OXFORD HANDBOO⸱ ⸱ NOV

Series Editors   R. N. Illingw⸱

OXFORD HANDBOOKS IN EMERGENCY MEDICINE

This series has already established itself as the essential reference series for staff in A & E departments.

Each book begins with an introduction to the topic, including epidemiology where appropriate. The clinical presentation and the immediate practical management of common conditions are described in detail, enabling the casualty officer or nurse to deal with the problem on the spot. Where appropriate a specific course of action is recommended for each situation and alternatives discussed. Information is clearly laid out and easy to find – important for situations where swift action may be vital.

Details of when, how, and to whom to refer patients are covered, as well as the information required at referral, and what this information is used for. The management of the patient after referral to a specialist is also outlined.

The text of each book is supplemented with checklists, key points, clear diagrams illustrating practical procedures, and recommendations for further reading.

The Oxford Handbooks in Emergency Medicine are an invaluable resource for every member of the A & E team, written and edited by clinicians at the sharp end.

Emergencies in Obstetrics and Gynaecology

Lindsey Stevens

Consultant/Honorary Senior Lecturer in
Accident and Emergency Medicine,
St. George's Hospital, London

in collaboration with:

Anthony Kenney

Consultant in Obstetrics and Gynaecology/
Honorary Senior Lecturer
St. Thomas' Hospital, London

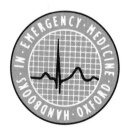

Oxford • New York • Tokyo
OXFORD UNIVERSITY PRESS
1994

Oxford University Press, Walton Street, Oxford OX2 6DP
Oxford   New York   Toronto
Delhi   Bombay   Calcutta   Madras   Karachi
Kuala Lumpur   Singapore   Hong Kong   Tokyo
Nairobi   Dar es Salaam   Cape Town
Melbourne   Auckland
and associated companies in
Berlin   Ibadan

Oxford is a trade mark of Oxford University Press

Published in the United States
by Oxford University Press Inc., New York

A catalogue record for this book is available from the British Library

Library of Congress Cataloging in Publication Data
Stevens, Lindsey.
Emergencies in obstetrics and gynaecology / Lindsey Stevens in
collaboration with Anthony Kenney.
(Oxford handbooks in emergency medicine ; 8)
Includes bibliographical references and index.
1. Obstetrical emergencies—Handbooks, manuals, etc.
2. Gynecologic emergencies—Handbooks, manuals, etc. I. Kenney,
Anthony. II. Title. III. Series.
[DNLM: 1. Genital Diseases, Female—handbooks. 2. Obstetrics—
handbooks. 3. Emergencies—handbooks. 4. Pregnancy Complications—
handbooks. WB 39 098 v.8 1994]
RG571.S83   1994   618'.0425—dc20   93–49710

ISBN 0 19 262470 9 (Hbk)
ISBN 0 19 262051 7 (Pbk)

Typeset by Footnote Graphics, Warminster, Wiltshire
Printed in Great Britain by
Biddles Ltd, Guildford & King's Lynn

Preface

One in twenty of all the patients attending our Accident and Emergency Departments have an obstetric or gynaecological complaint. Many of these cases are fraught with difficulty in that the diagnosis is unclear, but the possibility exists of life-threatening underlying pathology. Others of them present *in extremis*, and hesitant initial management of their resuscitation can end in fetal death or hypoxic damage, and in maternal morbidity or mortality. Some present in labour where mismanagement can convert a happy event into a tragedy.

The Report on Confidential Enquiries into Maternal Deaths 1985–87, judged that 84 out of the 115 women, who died from conditions directly related to pregnancy and birth, had received substandard care.

Pregnant women also come to the department with the same illnesses and injuries as affect the non-pregnant population. However, the expression of their condition is altered by the physiological and anatomical changes which accompany pregnancy, and their treatment often needs modification to take account of these changes and the safety of the fetus.

Few of the staff working in Accident and Emergency departments have previous specialist experience in Obstetrics and Gynaecology, and few obstetric staff are comfortable with the management of emergency cases such as the multiply injured patient.

This handbook, therefore, aims to provide guidance on the management of obstetric and gynaecological emergencies and on acute illness and injury affecting the pregnant patient for both groups of staff.

The guidance on emergency obstetric techniques is fairly comprehensive for, whilst most of the emergency departments in this country have immediate access to obstetric specialist help, there are still units without on-site obstetric care. Similarly, whilst brief reference is made to investigative techniques which may be provided in some centres, the text suggests radiological and laboratory techniques which are routinely available.

The handbook also covers the social and forensic aspects of assault, and legal issues as they affect gynaecological and obstetric practice in the emergency department. Guidance on the care and resuscitation of the new-born infant is included.

Background information is provided on anatomy, physiology, and drug prescription in pregnancy and a list of support organizations to which patients may be referred is appended.

The further reading suggested at the end of each chapter provides both more extensive coverage of the topic covered by the text and references to research work.

We hope that the book will be of use to medical and nursing staff in both emergency and obstetric and gynaecological practice. Primary care staff, general surgeons and physicians will also find sections relevant to their practice.

London   L.S.
June 1994   A.K.

Acknowledgements

Our thanks go to several colleagues at St. George's Health-care for their kind advice on sections of this book. Dr Fiona Davidson advised on Chapters 4 and 5, Dr Patricia Hamilton on Chapter 15, and Drs Parker-Williams, Wansborough-Jones, Eastwood, Millard, Maxwell, Wilson, Pumphrey, and Pearce on Chapter 10.

Anne Viney of Victim Support and Nicola Harwin of Women's Aid kindly reviewed the section on domestic violence, and Dr Frances Lewington, Head of the Forensic Medical Service, advised on the management of the rape victim.

The material contained in Appendix 2 is reproduced from the British National Formulary (25) by kind permission of the Royal Pharmaceutical Society of Great Britain and the British Medical Association.

Contents

x • Contents

PART 1
Basic principles of the assessment of the patient with a gynaecological or obstetric complaint

1 History and examination

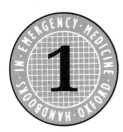

CHAPTER 1

History and examination

Key points in history and examination

1 The patient with early pregnancy may deny amenorrhoea but describe a change of menstrual pattern—careful questioning is mandatory.

2 Vaginal examination is contraindicated in ante-partum haemorrhage until an ultrasound scan has excluded placenta praevia. Vaginal examination should be limited to the use of a speculum when the clinical picture suggests an ectopic pregnancy.

3 The assessment of vaginal bleeding commences with a careful evaluation of the severity of haemorrhage.

4 Pain from pelvic viscera is poorly localized, being transmitted by the autonomic system to lower thoracic and upper lumbar roots.

5 The history of the patient presenting with vaginal discharge includes asking about the presence of genito-urinary symptoms in her partner.

6 Irradiation of the fetus should be minimized by careful selection of the imaging technique used, but the life of mother or fetus must never be endangered by the withholding of radiological investigations when these are needed to decide management.

Women who present to the Emergency Department with gynaecological or obstetric pathology may be broadly grouped into those presenting with bleeding *per vaginam*, those presenting with abdominal pain, and those presenting with vaginal discharge. This chapter first outlines a general approach and then aspects of the history and examination which are germane to these symptom groups. Childhood gynaecological illness or injury presents particular difficulties, and the history and examination of the young patient are considered in Chapter 6.

General history and examination

• **History   Examination**

History

When a patient presents with a complaint which seems primarily referable to the reproductive tract the general history should include the points in Box 1.1.

When **the patient is suspected or known to be pregnant** general symptoms of pregnancy should be sought, including nausea and vomiting (noting the frequency and amount of the latter), breast tenderness, and frequency of micturition. A brief history of antenatal care should be taken, noting where the patient is booked for delivery, what investigations have been performed in the antenatal clinic and the results of these, and any problems identified antenatally. The mother should be asked whether she has felt fetal movements and if so the last time that she was aware of them. If she is presenting post-partum a brief history of the labour and delivery should be taken, including whether labour was induced or spontaneous, its length, and any difficulties experienced during labour; the use of drugs, including syntocinon and anaesthetic agents; the method of delivery; and whether doubt was expressed about the completeness of the placenta. The mother should be asked about the number, gestational age, and state at birth of the child(ren) delivered, and about any problem identified post-partum, including genital tract trauma.

Box 1.1 **Points to be covered in history-taking**

Reproductive history
- Age of menarche
- Length of, and duration of bleeding in, usual menstrual cycle, regularity of the cycle, first day of last menses
- Whether sexually active; contraception used; any infective symptoms in partner
- Whether pregnancy is suspected by the patient; results of any pregnancy tests performed
- Number of previous pregnancies and outcome (miscarriage, termination, still or live birth)
- Age, birth weight, delivery method, and gestational age at birth of each child; cause of stillbirth
- Any previous antenatal, labour, or postnatal problems
- Gestational age of each fetus lost at, and any complications of, each miscarriage
- Method of each termination, stage, reason, and complications
- Age of menopause, peri-menopausal symptoms, post-menopausal problems (for example dyspareunia, bleeding)
- Any gynaecological operations or instrumentation
- Any sexual assault or abuse, past or present

General medical history
- Details of any serious illnesses or operations
- Systematic review of urinary system, including frequency, dysuria, haematuria, urgency, stress incontinence
- Systematic review of gastro-intestinal system, including alteration in bowel habit, blood loss *per rectum*

The assessing doctor must also enquire whether the child(ren) is(are) breast- or bottle-fed, as this will affect the prescription of treatment for the mother.

The general health survey should include enquiry regarding diabetes; hypertension; blood group, and history of blood transfusions; exposure to infections, including HepB/HIV risk; and drug usage (including smoking and alcohol)

Other history can usefully include the family history, for example of twins, diabetes, and hypertension; and the patient's social circumstances and relationship with her partner or family.

Examination

Whether or not vaginal examination is routinely performed by the Accident and Emergency doctor assessing the patient is a matter for local discussion and policy. Some practitioners believe that if patients require pelvic examination in the Emergency Department they will almost inevitably require referral to a gynaecologist, and vaginal examination should therefore be delayed until the gynaecologist arrives. There are other practitioners who would regard such delay as potentially dangerous. There are also Emergency Departments which do not have obstetric services on site. It is certainly true that intimate examinations should be kept to the safe minimum, and conducted with due regard for the comfort and dignity of the patient.

Vaginal examination is contraindicated when the patient has presented with antepartum haemorrhage. As palpation of the suspected ectopic has been known to lead to rupture, digital or bimanual examination is unwise when the history, abdominal examination, and pregnancy test suggest an ectopic pregnancy. A speculum examination is followed by ultrasound or laparoscopy as indicated in these patients.

The examination should commence with an overall impression of the patient whilst taking the history, and then limited **general examination**, including urinalysis (an empty bladder will be needed for abdominal and vaginal examinations), signs of anaemia, markers of pregnancy, blood pressure, pulse, chest, and breasts. Darkening of the areolae and the expression of fluid from the breasts are only useful indicators in the first pregnancy.

Abdominal examination should precede vaginal examination. Rectal examination follows if indicated.

The **abdominal examination** is performed with the bladder empty and the patient in the dorsal position, or in the lateral position if she cannot relax lying on her back. The usual sequence of inspection, palpation, percussion, and auscultation is followed.

During the inspection stretch marks, pigmentation, scars, and midline or flank fullness are of particular relevance.

Tumours felt on palpation should be assessed for position, size, shape, hardness, and mobility. Pelvic tumours are characteristically fixed in the cranio-caudal plane and mobile laterally; cysts may exhibit a fluid thrill. Many tumours are discovered incidentally during the course of examination for some other purpose, and the insidious nature and high mortality of ovarian carcinoma (4000 deaths p.a. in the UK) make assessment of the ovarian size a mandatory screening when patients are attending with a gynaecological concern. The ovaries should be impalpable after the menopause. Other presenting features of ovarian masses include abdominal distension, frequency of urination, retention, loin pain, change of bowel habit, venous thrombosis in the legs, cachexia, and general malaise.

Examination may reveal the cystic or solid nature of the tumour and the regularity of its surface. Mobility is an indicator of benign disease.

Ascites is associated with certain ovarian tumours, and should be sought on percussion where there is flank fullness or a pelvic tumour. An assessment of uterine size must be made; an enlarged uterus may be due to pregnancy, fibromyomata, uterine malignancy, or choriocarcinoma.

In early pregnancy the uterus will feel enlarged and softened, often with the body appearing softer than the cervix. As gestation progresses the cervix will also soften (by 16 weeks) and take on a bluish tinge. Fetal movements, parts, and heartbeat are usually palpable or audible by 26 weeks. The size of the uterus is related to the gestational age of the fetus, as is shown in Fig. 1.1. After the size of the uterus is estimated the examiner should feel the uterine lower pole to

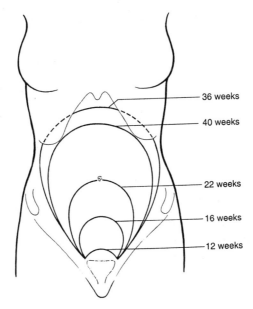

Fig. 1.1 • Change in fundal height during gestation.

assess lie and engagement. Subsequently the upper pole and sides are assessed.

On auscultation a uterine 'souffle' may be heard from the increased vascularity in the pregnant uterus or a large fibroid, and the fetal heart may be audible.

The **vaginal examination follows the sequence of**:

• Vulval inspection

• Inspection of the vagina and cervix

• Palpation of the vagina and cervix

• Bimanual examination

Whilst it is common practice to examine the patient in the dorsal position, it should be remembered that the lateral and Sims' positions are more acceptable to most patients and afford easier introduction of the speculum and a better view of the cervix and anterior vaginal wall. The abdominal muscles may also be more relaxed in these positions. The dorsal position should be used for bimanual palpation. Either a Sims' or a Cusco's speculum may be used for inspecting the vagina and cervix, the former giving a better view of the anterior vaginal wall and the latter of the cervix. A non-antiseptic gel is used for lubrication. Full antiseptic technique is, however, mandatory for any patient who may be in labour or have ruptured membranes. Any discharge is assessed by taking endocervical swabs and slides as indicated in Box 1.2, p. 15. A cervical smear should be taken using an Ayres spatula. Material should be collected from both the posterior fornix and the cervix. Care should be taken to include the squamo-columnar junction, the longer portion of the spatula blade being placed in the external os and the blade rotated across the whole cervical surface. The smear must be immediately spread on a slide and placed in fixative.

The speculum is then removed and palpation of the vaginal walls, fornices, and cervix is performed using the gloved index finger. The position and direction of the cervix should be noted, as well as its surface and the shape of the external os.

Finally, bimanual palpation is performed, using two gloved fingers in the vagina, with the other hand on the lower abdomen. Where the uterus is anteverted, the vaginal fingers should be placed in the anterior fornix; the uterus can then be palpated between the two hands. Where cervical assessment has indicated that the uterus is retroverted, the vaginal fingers should be placed in the posterior fornix. The uterine size, shape, position, mobility, and tenderness are noted. Next the examining fingers are placed in the lateral fornices, and the adnexa examined. The fallopian tubes may be felt if they are thickened, but are not normally palpable. The ovary may be felt as a 4 cm by 2 cm mobile, slightly tender mass, but is usually impalpable unless the patient is thin.

Rectal examination may be needed to elucidate suspected abnormalities in the rectovaginal pouch or the uterosacral or broad ligaments.

Aspects specific to common complaints

- The patient presenting with vaginal bleeding   The patient presenting with abdominal pain   The patient presenting with vaginal discharge

The patient presenting with vaginal bleeding

Vaginal examination is contraindicated for patients in the third trimester who present with vaginal bleeding until ultrasonography has excluded a placenta praevia. Digital vaginal examination is unwise when an ectopic pregnancy is suspected on the history and abdominal examination.

The history should include the amount of bleeding (including towel or tampon usage), the passage of clots or other material, and the pattern of bleeding, particularly its relationship to menses. There may be associated symptoms such as dyspareunia or pelvic pain. Particular and detailed attention must be given to the possibility that the patient is in the early stages of pregnancy. The patient with early pregnancy may deny amenorrhoea but describe a change of menstrual pattern both in quantity and timing of bleeding over the two or three months preceding presentation; careful questioning is therefore mandatory. Where there is any possibility of pregnancy a urine HCG test must be performed. There may be associated coagulopathy, and history and examination should cover bleeding and bruising tendencies. The severity of haemorrhage must be carefully assessed by pulse rate, blood pressure, respiratory rate, and urine output measurements performed repeatedly. These measurements can be used to gauge the amount of probable blood/fluid loss (see Table 1.1).

The assessment of the pregnant patient is significantly altered by the changes in respiratory and cardiovascular function which accompany pregnancy (see Box 11.1, p. 151) and the patient's resuscitation must be adapted to allow for these changes. The pregnant woman near term may lose up to 35 per cent of her circulating volume before exhibiting the signs of shock, cushioning the loss by shunting blood away from the utero-placental circulation. The fetus, by contrast, is compromised as soon as this shunting starts. The assessing physician must estimate blood loss on the basis of the history and commence high-flow oxygen and intravenous fluids for any pregnant woman with other than trivial bleeding. Blood transfusion should be started relatively early in the resuscitation. Central venous pressure monitoring is a useful guide to the response to fluid resuscitation in the pregnant patient.

Where it is estimated that the patient has lost up to 750 ml of her blood volume, the infusion of crystalloid solution to restore the intravascular volume should suffice; above this degree of bleeding blood transfusion should be arranged. Where bleeding is brisk or the blood loss is thought to exceed 1500 ml, type-specific blood transfusion should be instituted as soon as possible. Where the patient is clinically shocked or bleeding is profuse, transfusion with blood group O Rhesus negative blood should be commenced.

The pregnant woman may become hypotensed by decreased venous return from the compression of the inferior vena cava by the gravid uterus (supine hypotension). This should be avoided by nursing the patient on her left side or by elevating the right buttock and displacing the uterus to the left manually.

Table 1.1 • Estimated blood/fluid loss for average adult based on initial observations

Pulse rate	<100	>100	>120	>140
Blood pressure	Normal	Normal	Low	Low
Pulse pressure	Normal	Decreased	Decreased	Decreased
Urine (mls/hr)	over 30	20–30	5–15	minimal
Respiratory rate	14–20	20–30	30–40	over 35
Blood loss (in l)	Up to 0.75	0.75–1.5	1.5–2.0	over 2.0

Examination includes an assessment of uterine size (see Fig. 1.1, p. 9). Undue enlargement may indicate uterine carcinoma or gestational trophoblastic disease; a uterus which is unexpectedly small for the gestational dates may be an indicator of an ectopic pregnancy or a missed abortion.

During examination a careful search should be made for vulval, vaginal, or cervical lesions which may be the origin of the blood loss. Products of conception may be seen lying in the external os. These may cause profound hypotension due to a vagal effect, and may need immediate intervention (see Chapter 8).

If no local lesion is seen, there is no blood passing through the cervical os, and the os is closed, the possibility that the bleeding originated from the urinary tract or rectum should lead to evaluation of these structures.

The patient presenting with abdominal pain

In differentiating between the causes of abdominal pain the patient should be asked whether there is a possibility of pregnancy, whether the onset was acute or gradual, the characteristics (site, degree, duration, nature) of the pain, whether the pattern of the pain can be related to the menstrual cycle, whether sexual intercourse is painful, and whether there are other precipitating or relieving factors, and/or associated symptoms such as vaginal bleeding.

An abrupt onset of pain suggests rupture, perforation, torsion, or haemorrhage into a cyst. A slower onset suggests inflammation or obstruction. A steady pain suggests inflammation; a colicky pain distension of a hollow viscus. Pain that is exacerbated by movement suggests peritoneal irritation from inflammation rather than obstruction of a viscus. Syncope should suggest haemorrhage.

Whilst pain from the vulva, perineum, and lower vagina is well localized, sensation being transmitted via the pudendal nerves to the second, third, and fourth sacral roots, that from the pelvic viscera is poorly localized, being transmitted by the autonomic system to roots at lower thoracic and upper lumbar level. Figure 1.2 indicates the localization of pain arising from the intra-abdominal organs. Much of the awareness of pathology in the viscera is due to irritation of the overlying peritoneum or to the effect of intraperitoneal bleeding. The pain associated with a haemoperitoneum is aching and constant, may be referred to the shoulder-tip, and may be associated with the signs and symptoms of hypovolaemia.

Backache may accompany gynaecological disease, but is a much rarer manifestation than is generally thought. Characteristically such pain is of gradual onset, felt below the level of T10, and not associated with pain radiating down the leg,

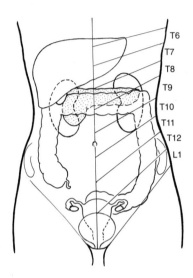

Fig. 1.2 • The localization of abdominal pain. Afferent visceral impulses by dermatome.

movement, or local tenderness. However, the possibility of sciatic nerve entrapment as a result of cervical carcinoma or bony metastases must be remembered.

During physical examination, the deportment of the patient may indicate the source of pain. Patients with pancreatitis or appendicitis are often more comfortable on their sides with the knees bent. Colicky pains such as that from torsion may cause restlessness. When peritonitis is present movement is painful and the patient lies very still. During palpation peritonism should be carefully sought. Cervical excitation accompanies peritonism from any cause. The finding of a palpable mass on examination is a helpful pointer, and should be methodically sought.

The patient presenting with vaginal discharge

The history should include enquiry into the amount, colour, and odour of the discharge, into recent sexual contacts and symptoms experienced by such recent sexual contacts, and into accompanying symptoms, such as vulval soreness or irritation, dyspareunia, or vaginal bleeding.

Normal vaginal discharge is a clear or white mixture of cervical mucus, endometrial gland secretion, vaginal transudate, and desquamated epithelial cells. It increases at ovulation, premenstrually, and during pregnancy. The multiplication of pathogenic bacteria is inhibited by the acid pH caused by the conversion of glycogen in the fluid to lactic acid by Doderlein's bacilli.

Examination should commence with careful inspection of the vulva for local lesions. During vulval inspection the examiner notes any discharge and its characteristics, and then examines the labia, clitoris, the orifices of Bartholin's ducts, and the urethral orifice. The urethra is examined for discharge by using a finger in the vagina to compress it from behind forwards. The patient is then assessed for stress incontinence by being asked to cough.

Vaginal examination may show punctate reddening and bleeding from infective vaginitis or the smooth pink appearance of atrophic vaginitis. The cervix should also be carefully inspected for cervicitis and for discharge or bleeding passing through the cervical os.

Specimens of the discharge should be taken for laboratory examination as indicated in Box 1.2.

Box 1.2 **The laboratory evaluation of vaginal discharge requires:**

- Wet slide preparation
- Swab for *Trichomonas vaginalis* in specialist transport medium
- Swab for *Candida*, aerobes, anaerobes in Stuart's medium
- Swab for *Gonococcus* in charcoal medium (or, best, plated immediately on to chocolate agar)
- Swab for *Chlamydia* in chlamydial specialist transport medium
- Cervical smear slide in fixative

Note: Where TV medium is not available, swabs may be placed in Stuart's medium.

Imaging techniques

Specific comments about the usefulness of imaging investigations are made in relation to the main topics of each chapter in this book. However, certain general points are noteworthy. Firstly, radiological examinations should be minimized in the pregnant patient, both in number and in the component parts of each test. Indeed, they should be employed cautiously in any woman of reproductive age, every effort being made to elicit a history of possible pregnancy before tests are ordered. It is a wise general precaution to protect uterus and ovaries routinely with a lead guard. Fluoroscopic examinations expose the patient to far higher radiation than simple films. Consideration should always be given to using some other form of imaging; but, above all, it is vital never to endanger the life of mother or fetus by withholding radiological investigations where these are needed to decide management.

Ultrasonic examination may be performed either transabdominally or using a vaginal probe. The latter technique has enhanced the ability to view the ovaries, recto-vaginal pouch, and uterus. The fetal sac is visible in most pregnancies at five weeks after the last menstrual period.

Further reading

Levitt, M. A. (1991). An evaluation of clinical variables in determining the need for pelvic examination in the emergency department. *Annals of emergency medicine*, **20** (4), 351–4.

PART 2
The assessment and management of the patient where pregnancy is not suspected

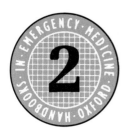

CHAPTER 2

The non-pregnant patient presenting with bleeding *per vaginam*

Key points in the non-pregnant patient presenting with bleeding *per vaginam*

1 As with all cases of haemorrhage presenting to the emergency department, the first priority is the assessment, resuscitation, and stabilization of the patient.

2 Severe anaemia may result from prolonged bleeding. The haemoglobin level should be noted and iron therapy, or transfusion, offered as indicated.

3 No patient with a continuing haemorrhagic problem should be lost to follow up. It is the responsibility of the assessing physician to ensure that appropriate out-patient care is arranged if the patient is fit to discharge from the emergency department.

4 Peri-menopausal patients presenting with vaginal bleeding must not be commenced on hormonal treatment before neoplasia has been excluded.

5 The possibility of toxic shock syndrome should be considered in any woman of reproductive age presenting with pyrexia, hypotension, and a rash.

6 The natural history of cervical carcinoma means that deaths from this cause are avoidable. A cervical smear should be taken in A and E where the appearance of the cervix is unusual, there is a discharge or post-coital bleeding, or the cervix bleeds on examination. Follow-up of the results of these smears must be ensured.

General points

- **Differential diagnosis of bleeding *per vaginam***

As with all cases of haemorrhage presenting to the emergency department, the first priority is the assessment and stabilization of the patient. Blood-pressure and pulse-rate observations must be repeated at regular intervals, and an estimate of the amount of bleeding charted. Where the bleeding is of significant extent intravenous fluids must be commenced and baseline measurements of the full blood count and clotting profile, as well as blood grouping, ordered. Secondly, it should be remembered that severe anaemia may result from prolonged bleeding, and the haemoglobin level should be measured and iron therapy or transfusion offered as indicated. Thirdly, no patient with a continuing haemorrhagic problem should be lost to follow-up. It is the responsibility of the assessing physician to ensure that appropriate outpatient care is arranged if the patient is fit to discharge from the emergency department. Gynaecological referral should be made where there is continuous or irregular bleeding even if a local lesion is found, as there may be a coexisting carcinoma. Boxes 2.1 and 2.2 detail the approach to the patient.

Bleeding related to the menstrual cycle

- **Dysfunctional uterine bleeding (DUB)   Endometriosis Uterine fibromyomata ('fibroids')   Toxic shock syndrome**

Dysfunctional uterine bleeding is defined as heavy (menorrhagia) or irregular (polymenorrhoea, metrorrhagia) bleeding where no local cause is found and there is no pregnancy. The dysfunction is caused by alterations in the output of, or balance between, ovarian hormones, gonadotrophins, and uterine prostaglandins.

The menstrual cycles of women with dysfunctional bleeding may be ovular or anovular. In ovulatory cycles the corpus luteum may underproduce oestrogen and progesterone,

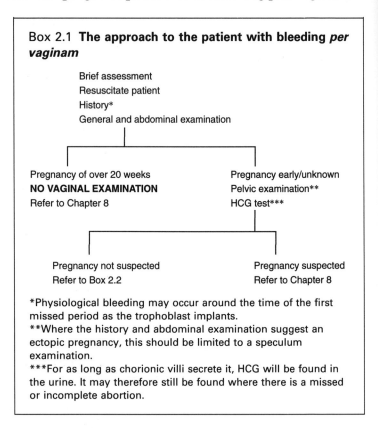

Box 2.1 **The approach to the patient with bleeding *per vaginam***

Brief assessment
Resuscitate patient
History*
General and abdominal examination

Pregnancy of over 20 weeks
NO VAGINAL EXAMINATION
Refer to Chapter 8

Pregnancy early/unknown
Pelvic examination**
HCG test***

Pregnancy not suspected
Refer to Box 2.2

Pregnancy suspected
Refer to Chapter 8

*Physiological bleeding may occur around the time of the first missed period as the trophoblast implants.
**Where the history and abdominal examination suggest an ectopic pregnancy, this should be limited to a speculum examination.
***For as long as chorionic villi secrete it, HCG will be found in the urine. It may therefore still be found where there is a missed or incomplete abortion.

giving a short luteal phase accompanied by an irregular endometrial response. In other cases the luteal phase may be long, with abnormal persistence of the corpus luteum, sometimes as a luteal cyst. In anovular cycles the oestrogen level rises, follicle stimulating hormone (FSH) is inhibited by the oestrogen feedback loop, the oestrogen level falls, and the endometrium is shed. Dysfunctional bleeding may be the presenting feature of infertility.

The uterine endometrium relatively underproduces prostaglandin F2α (PGF2α) and overproduces prostaglandin E2 (PGE2) in some cases of dysfunctional bleeding.

In some cases there is cystic glandular hyperplasia due to the absence of a negative feedback effect on the hypothalamus of the initial oestrogen rise of the menstrual cycle. FSH

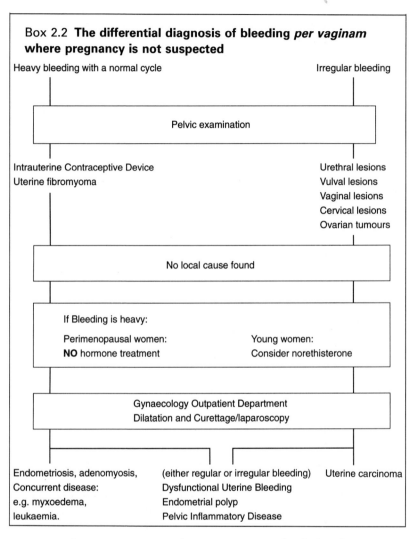

Box 2.2 **The differential diagnosis of bleeding *per vaginam* where pregnancy is not suspected**

Heavy bleeding with a normal cycle
Irregular bleeding

Pelvic examination

Intrauterine Contraceptive Device
Uterine fibromyoma

Urethral lesions
Vulval lesions
Vaginal lesions
Cervical lesions
Ovarian tumours

No local cause found

If Bleeding is heavy:

Perimenopausal women:
NO hormone treatment

Young women:
Consider norethisterone

Gynaecology Outpatient Department
Dilatation and Curettage/laparoscopy

Endometriosis, adenomyosis,
Concurrent disease:
e.g. myxoedema,
leukaemia.

(either regular or irregular bleeding)
Dysfunctional Uterine Bleeding
Endometrial polyp
Pelvic Inflammatory Disease

Uterine carcinoma

and oestrogen secretion continue at high levels, causing amenorrhoea and endometrial hyperplasia. Bleeding occurs either when portions of the excessively thick endometrium outgrow their blood supply or as the oestrogen level begins to fluctuate with time.

Post-menarche menorrhagia may be due to anovular cycles or to endometrial hyperplasia from oestrogen action in the absence of progesterone. The effect of emotion on menstrual pattern and flow is thought to be due to the hypothalamic–pituitary axis response to higher centres. This may lie behind the change of pattern which may accompany a change of country and climate. Short menstrual cycles may be due to inadequate ovarian or corpus luteal function. They may be found after childbirth or abortion.

Nearly all cases of dysfunctional bleeding around puberty recover spontaneously. Unless there are specific indications in the history, curettage is unnecessary. If the bleeding is excessive, norethisterone may be used (a reducing regime over ten days commencing at 5 mg three times a day). Irregular or heavy bleeding around the menopause *must* be fully investigated with curettage. Hysterectomy may be offered in preference to prolonged hormonal treatment.

During the child-bearing years, an expectant policy may be pursued initially. Where bleeding is significant, the emergency physician may commence norethisterone 5 mg three times a day for 5 days as a holding measure while the patient awaits her outpatient appointment. Curettage should be offered whenever the period of abnormal bleeding has exceeded three months or the flow is excessive. Where an anovular cycle pattern is indicated histologically norethisterone 5 mg twice a day from day 16 to day 25 of the cycle may be of benefit. Alternatively, a combined oestrogen–progestogen pill may be used for 21 out of 28 days. Cyclooxygenase inhibitors such as mefanamic acid are unpredictable in their effects, but may be valuable regulators of the uterine prostaglandin production.

Antifibrinolytics such as tranexamic acid may be of use, as may danazol. Where medical treatment has failed to control the bleeding, endometrial ablation with a laser or electrosurgery has been found to be effective. Finally, hysterectomy with preservation of the ovaries may have to be offered.

Anaemia and iron therapy, or occasionally transfusion, may be indicated. Lastly the effect of the inconvenience attendant on menstrual irregularities on the patient's life and psyche should not be underestimated.

Endometriosis is defined as the existence of endometrium in locations other than the innermost layer of the uterus.

Areas of endometriosis located intramurally in the uterus are called adenomyosis. The sites affected are listed in Box 2.3.

Box 2.3 Endometriosis. Sites ranked by incidence

- ovarian
- rectovaginal
- uterine wall
- uterosacral ligaments
- pelvic peritoneum applied to for example bowel, bladder, or fallopian tube
- umbilical
- vulval
- inguinal
- in abdominal wall scars

The islets of endometriosis show typical endometrial glands and stroma. The tissue follows the changes of the menstrual cycle, including bleeding, which may give rise to brown-fluid-filled cysts (for example the ovarian 'chocolate cyst'). Cystic hyperplasia may be found. Adhesions form around the affected areas. The pathological origins of this condition are unclear. Theories include (a) metaplasia of the peritoneal endothelial cells; (b) spill of live fragments of endometrium into the peritoneal cavity during menstruation and their implantation and growth; and (c) in adenomyosis, downgrowth from the endometrium into the myometrium (reason unknown).

Women of low parity, late to bear children, or of Caucasian origin are particularly at risk. There is a familial tendency.

Endometriosis appears after puberty, regresses during pregnancy, and clears with the menopause.

The main symptoms of endometriosis are pelvic pain, dysmenorrhoea, dyspareunia, and abnormal uterine bleeding. Alternatively endometriosis may be found incidentally at operation or during the course of investigation for infertility (30–50 per cent of endometriosis sufferers are infertile). The patient may present with severe acute abdominal pain where a cyst has ruptured into the peritoneal cavity, or with rectal pain and/or bleeding *per rectum* at the time of menstruation where there is rectal involvement. Bladder endometriosis can present as frequency or haematuria accompanying menstruation. On examination endometriosis may be manifest externally in scar tissue or the umbilicus. There may be a fixed cystic tumour in the rectovaginal pouch where there is ovarian involvement, moderate uterine enlargement where adenomyosis is a feature of the disease, a tender indurated mass palpable *per rectum* where there is involvement of the rectovaginal septum, or the signs of intestinal obstruction where the bowel is affected. Vaginal endometriosis may be visible on speculum examination.

Serum markers have been identified for endometriosis, but the specificity of the present markers is too low for their use as a screening test. Ultrasound is of limited usefulness, and laparoscopy remains the diagnostic test of choice. Treatment is hormonal or surgical. Lesions can be excised or coagulated by laser or cautery if small. The extent of surgical clearance should be adjusted to the patient's desire for children. Hormonal therapy is directed at suppression of the menstrual cycle by high-dose progesterone, androgens (for example danazol, gestrinone) and GnRH agonists which suppress FSH and LH (for example buserelin, goserelin). The recurrence rate on stopping therapy is high.

Uterine fibromyomata ('fibroids') are composed of smooth muscle and fibrous tissue arranged in whorled bundles and separated by a capsule of loose connective tissue from the myometrium. The centre of the tumour may degenerate as it outstrips its blood supply, the tissue undergoing hyaline or cystic change. Fatty degeneration also occurs; where this is followed by renewal of the blood supply 'red' degeneration ensues. Calcification occurs in the elderly. Some 98 per cent of fibroids arise in the body of the uterus. As they grow they tend to be extruded towards the cavity or the peritoneum. Subendometrial fibroids may be pushed into the cervix by uterine contractions and appear as polyps. Subperitoneal fibroids may become pedunculated, mimicking an ovarian tumour and becoming liable to tort. Torsion, infection of a necrotic area, and malignant change may occur. The incidence of malignancy is 0.2 per cent, the type usually being a spindle cell sarcoma.

Pregnancy and oestrogen-containing contraceptive pills encourage growth of these tumours, and they may atrophy at the menopause. They are more common in the nulliparous, those women with no recent pregnancy, and Afro-Caribbeans.

Fibromyomata may present with menorrhagia, the patient's or attending physician's discovery of a lump, abdominal discomfort, or, rarely, pain where there is attempted extrusion *per vaginam*. There may be symptoms of accompanying distortion of the urethra, such as frequency or retention, perhaps with a menstrual cyclicity. Red degeneration may present with pain, enlargement, and tenderness, torsion with acute abdominal pain and shock, infection with tenderness and an offensive discharge, and malignancy with irregular bleeding and rapid growth. Systemic symptoms such as pyrexia and vomiting may accompany these secondary changes.

Surgical removal by myomectomy or hysterectomy is indicated where there is heavy bleeding, urinary symptoms, torsion, interference with pregnancy, possible malignancy, or large size.

Fibroids may cause infertility or spontaneous abortion. Pregnancy progresses uneventfully in most cases. Red degeneration may occur and may be treated conservatively with pain-relief and rest. Where the fibroid is low and will obstruct labour Caesarean hysterectomy is indicated.

Hyperplastic change in endometrium and myometrium, ovarian follicular cysts, and pelvic endometriosis are associated with this condition. Endometrial carcinoma has been found at operation for fibroids, and salpingitis is also a common association (possibly because of shared patient demographic characteristics rather than pathology).

Finally, patients may present during the course of a menstrual period with **toxic shock syndrome.** The patient presents with pyrexia, diarrhoea, hypotensive shock, and an erythematous rash. The history given is of tampon use, particularly of those of the highly absorbent variety. Patients usually present between the second and fourth days of menstruation, and state that their illness began in the early morning. An exotoxin produced by *Staphylococcus aureus* is known to be sometimes responsible, and *Streptococcus* has also been implicated. The staphylococcal toxin is introduced into the bloodstream by breaks in the vaginal or cervical epithelium or by retrograde menstrual flow carrying it intraperitoneally. The condition is serious, renal failure may ensue, and deaths have occurred. Any tampon is removed, vaginal swabs are taken for culture, vaginal lavage is performed, and treatment with intravenous flucloxacillin is initiated.

Bleeding unrelated to menstruation

- **Urethral lesions   Carcinoma of the vagina   Cervical erosion   Cervical polyps   Cervical neoplastic change   Uterine endometrial polyps   Carcinoma of the body of the uterus   Fallopian tumour   Ovarian tumours**

Local lesions of the urethra, vulva, vagina, and cervix may be responsible for bleeding unrelated to menstruation.

Urethral lesions include caruncle, diverticulum, and carcinoma. The small, bright red swelling of a urethral caruncle arises from the posterior wall of the urethra. It may present with bleeding, dyspareunia, painful micturition, or tenderness, or may be asymptomatic. It is a benign granulomatous tumour, and is commoner post-menopause.

A urethral diverticulum presents as a vaginal wall swelling or with frequency and dysuria. There may be the passage of blood or pus *per urethram*.

Urethral carcinoma presents as a thickened area around the orifice. Bleeding is common and retention may occur.

Carcinoma of the vagina may present with postcoital bleeding, an offensive thin discharge, or urine or faeces *per vaginam*. Primary carcinoma is usually squamous, although adenocarcinomas have been found in the daughters of mothers treated with stilboestrol during pregnancy. There may be local spread from cervix or uterus or metastatic spread from uterus, ovary, or cervix.

Choriocarcinoma may metastasize to the vagina; it presents as a purplish nodule which bleeds easily. HCG levels will be high.

Cervical lesions include erosion, polyp, and neoplasia.

Cervical erosion is defined as the replacement of the stratified epithelium which covers the vaginal surface of the cervix with columnar epithelium. The junctional zone between squamous and columnar epithelium in the cervix is dynamic, with shift of the boundaries between the two types continuing at a low level all the time. The dominance of the columnar epithelium appears to be hormonally triggered, although the precise mechanism is unknown. Oral contraceptives, pregnancy, and delivery act as triggers for the condition. Patients present with a mucoid discharge. There may be postcoital or intermenstrual bleeding, or loss during pregnancy. **Such bleeding is always slight.** There is no pain or dyspareunia. On examination there is a red, rough area around the os.

No treatment is necessary as an emergency. Thermal, cryosurgical, or laser cautery are offered by the gynaecologists.

Cervical polyps originate from the endocervix and consist of mucus-producing cervical glands covered with columnar epithelium. They present with bleeding, often post-coital. On examination they appear as red or pink soft polyps depending from the external os, sometimes as far as the vaginal orifice. The polyp may be twisted off without anaesthesia; the result must be sent for histological examination, and the patient must be referred to gynaecological outpatients for re-evaluation and for cauterization of the stalk of the polyp, which may involve dilatation of the cervical canal under anaesthesia.

Cervical neoplastic change is characterized by a lack of differentiation of the cells, nuclear abnormalities, and increased mitoses. Three grades of pre-cancerous change are defined: CIN (cervical intraepithelial neoplasia) 1, 2, and 3.

Aetiological factors include intercourse from an early age and a large number of sexual partners. Human papilloma virus has been suggested as the carcinogen responsible.

Progression from one grade to the next is not inevitable. CIN1 may revert to normal, but 30 per cent of CIN3 cases progress to invasive carcinoma, although it is characteristic of this progression that it takes years.

Frank carcinoma is 90 per cent squamous, and 10 per cent columnar; 17 per cent of carcinoma arises in the cervical canal, and the rest on the ectocervix. The tumour spreads locally into the bladder, along the uterosacral ligaments, and towards the pelvic side-walls. Lymphatic spread occurs to the internal iliac and presacral nodes. Metastatic spread is rare, as death usually follows the effects of local invasion. The carcinoma is clinically staged from IB to IVB by the degree of local and distant involvement.

Cervical intraepithelial neoplasia is asymptomatic, and the cervix looks normal to the naked eye.

Patients with carcinoma present with postcoital bleeding, or bleeding associated with defecation or micturition. Later, bleeding becomes continuous, and a thin, bloody, increasingly offensive discharge develops. Carcinoma may block the internal os, giving rise to a pyometra. Pain is a late sign, signifying spread beyond the cervix; it may be felt in the lower abdomen or back (from uterosacral ligament or presacral node involvement), and may be severe and intractable. Back pain may also be due to vertebral metastases. As the bladder and rectum become involved, incontinence of urine and faeces supervenes, and vesicovaginal and rectovaginal fistulae occur. Ureteral obstruction and pyelonephritis occur, and the associated uraemia is the commonest cause of death.

On speculum examination, a nodule, ulcer, or 'erosion' may be seen, all of which are characteristically friable. Later the lesion may look warty, or crater-like. Endocervical carcinoma gives a firm, barrel-shaped cervix, which later ulcerates, giving a large central cavity. The mobility of the cervix is lost once there is local invasion; spread may be felt *per rectum*.

The natural history of cervical carcinoma means that deaths from this cause are avoidable. There are 2000 deaths per annum. Five-year survival at Stage 1 is over 85 per cent, but at Stage IV it is 5 per cent.

A cervical smear should be taken in A and E where the appearance of the cervix is unusual, there is a discharge or postcoital bleeding, or the cervix bleeds on examination. All women should have routine cervical smears at regular intervals. The present Department of Health recommendations are that women between the ages of 25 and 60 should have a cervical smear every three years.

There is a case for the performance of 'routine' smears in the A and E department where patients might otherwise escape the net. When taking a smear the sample must include cells from the ecto- and endocervix, as the transformation zone may lie in the cervical canal. Specimens must be immediately fixed in alcohol. Follow-up arrangements must be made to ensure that the result of the test catches up with the patient.

Where there is clinical suspicion of malignancy gynaecological referral must be made.

Bleeding through the cervical os may be due to uterine, fallopian, or ovarian tumours.

Uterine endometrial polyps are small, soft, red, collections of endometrium and glands. They may show cystic hyperplasia. They show the usual cyclical changes, and may present with menorrhagia or irregular bleeding.

Carcinoma of the body of the uterus is defined as carcinoma arising cranial to the internal os. The vast majority of tumours are adenocarcinomas, although squamous elements may occur. There may be spread to the urethra, vagina, cervix, ovaries, and intraperitoneal structures. Pulmonary, bony, or other metastases may appear; lymphatic spread is usually to the para-aortic nodes. The aetiological factors are outlined in Box 2.4.

Uterine carcinoma commonly presents with post-

Box 2.4 Aetiology of uterine carcinoma

- post-menopausal (75 per cent)
- oestrogen administration
- polycystic ovaries
- oestrogen-secreting ovarian tumours
- late menopause
- diabetes, hypertension, obesity

menopausal bleeding, which becomes increasingly heavy and frequent. Pre-menopausally, the pattern is one of irregular intermenstrual blood loss, which must not be mistaken for the onset of the menopause (menopausal menstrual loss becomes lighter or further apart, or stops altogether). There may be a thin discharge which becomes offensive. Pain is a late complaint.

The uterus may not feel enlarged, and there may be an apparent local lesion to account for the bleeding. It is, however, imperative that curettage should be carried out even in these circumstances, to rule out a co-existing carcinoma. Treatment is by hysterectomy and bilateral salpingo-oophorectomy, with further resection and adjuvant radiotherapy and progestogens as dictated by the staging of the carcinoma at laparotomy. Anaemia may be severe; otherwise the complications are those of the invasion of local pelvic structures or of metastatic spread.

The uterus may also give rise to sarcomatous and mesodermal tumours, which also present with bleeding. These grow quickly, with pain being a relatively early symptom. Local and metastatic spread is common, and the prognosis is poor. Treatment is by radical surgery, irradiation, and chemotherapy in selected cases.

Rarely a primary **fallopian tumour** may present with an intermittent bloodstained, thin discharge. Pain and ascites may be associated, an abdominal mass may be felt. Treatment is similar to that for uterine carcinoma.

Fuller details of **ovarian tumours** may be found in Chapter 3. The following paragraphs confine themselves to those neoplasias characteristically presenting with bleeding irregularities. Any ovarian malignancy may present with bleeding if it has eroded through into the uterus or vagina.

Corpus luteal cysts arise where there has been excessive bleeding into the follicle at the time of ovulation. They continue to secrete progesterone, and therefore delay menstruation beyond the normal life of the corpus luteum. The cyst may be tender to palpation. Menstruation is heavier than usual when it occurs.

Granulosa and theca cell tumours are defined as tumours derived from the granulosa cells of the follicle and the adjacent theca interna. The tumours are solid when small, and become cystic as they enlarge, which may be to a remarkable size. They have a high lipoid content, and are yellowish in cross-section. Tumours are bilateral in a significant proportion of cases. These growths are of low-grade malignancy. Local invasion, peritoneal seedlings, and lymphatic and blood-borne spread may occur, and metastases may be found, sometimes many years after surgical removal of the primary tumour. It is characteristic of both thecomata and granulosa cell tumours that they produce reproductive hormones. The vast majority are oestrogen-producing, although a few produce progesterone. Where levels of oestrogen are high menstruation is delayed and the endometrium hypertrophies. Ovulation is suppressed by feedback on the pituitary gland.

In young patients the tumour presents with precocious puberty (see Chapter 6), which may appear in emergency medicine practice as a complaint of bleeding *per vaginam*. Patients of reproductive age present with irregular, often heavy menstruation. Older patients present with postmenopausal bleeding. Endometrial carcinoma is associated with some 4 per cent of post-menopausal cases. The tumour may present with torsion at any age.

The tumour is staged at laparotomy; those cases where the growth appears to be limited to a single ovary and the patient wishes to have children may be treated with unilateral salpingo-oophorectomy. In all other cases total hysterectomy, bilateral salpingo-oophorectomy, and omentectomy are performed, followed by chemotherapy, usually with paraplatin.

Further reading

Dysfunctional uterine bleeding and menorrhagia (1989). *Baillière's Clinical Obstetrics and Gynaecology*, **3** (2), 217–424.

Lambert, H. E. and Blake, P. R. (eds) (1992). *Gynaecological oncology*, Oxford University Press, New York.

Magos, A. L. (1992). Transcervical endometrial ablation in the treatment of dysfunctional uterine bleeding. In *Recent advances* in *obstetrics and gynaecology*, Vol. 17 (ed. J. Bonnar), pp. 191–208. Churchill Livingstone, Edinburgh.

Naish, C. E. and Barlow, D. H. (1992). Endometriosis. *Hospital Update*, **18** (8), 598–606.

Smith, S. K. and Haining, R. E. B. (1992). The investigation and management of excessive menstrual bleeding. In *Recent advances in obstetrics and gynaecology*, Vol. 17 (ed. J. Bonnar), pp. 171–89, Churchill Livingstone, Edinburgh.

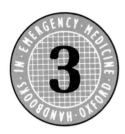

CHAPTER 3

The non-pregnant patient presenting with pelvic pain

Key points in the non-pregnant patient presenting with pelvic pain

1 The relationship of pain to the menstrual cycle, the pattern of onset of the pain and the presence of dyspareunia are useful pointers in the history.

2 Torsion of, rupture of, and haemorrhage into, an ovarian mass may all present with severe, acute iliac fossa pain. Torsion of an ovarian mass may, however, present with intermittent, colicky pain. Urgent laparotomy is essential when torsion has occurred.

3 The patient with ovarian hyperstimulation may present with hypotension and a tender mass in the iliac fossa mimicking ectopic pregnancy. However, the haematocrit is raised.

Patients presenting with pelvic pain of acute onset

- **Differential diagnosis of acute pelvic pain**

The approach to the differential diagnosis of acute pelvic pain when pregnancy is not suspected is summarized in Box 3.1.

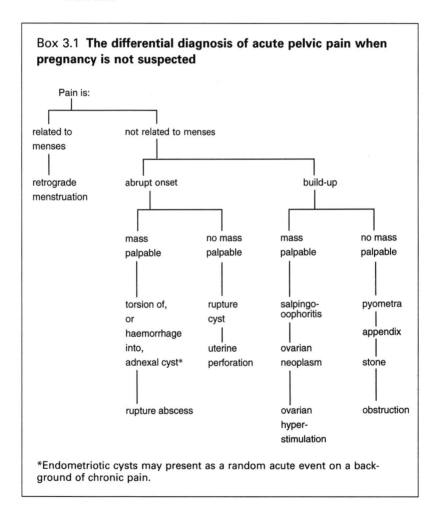

Box 3.1 The differential diagnosis of acute pelvic pain when pregnancy is not suspected

Pain is:

related to menses → retrograde menstruation

not related to menses:

- abrupt onset
  - mass palpable → torsion of, or haemorrhage into, adnexal cyst* → rupture abscess
  - no mass palpable → rupture cyst → uterine perforation
- build-up
  - mass palpable → salpingo-oophoritis → ovarian neoplasm → ovarian hyper-stimulation
  - no mass palpable → pyometra → appendix → stone → obstruction

*Endometriotic cysts may present as a random acute event on a background of chronic pain.

Pain accompanying the onset of menstruation, rather than preceding it, is characteristic of irritation of the peritoneum by **retrograde leakage of menstrual blood** from the fallopian tubes. Vaginal examination is mildly painful.

Enlargement of the ovary may result from benign functional cysts, primary ovarian cysts and tumours from the surface epithelium, germ cells, or sex cord or gonadal stroma, or from metastatic spread of non-ovarian malignancy. Of the non-neoplastic cysts, **follicular cysts** are by far the most common. They are granulosa cell-lined, fluid-containing cysts which may reach 5 cm in size and resolve spontaneously. Small ovarian masses are usually therefore simply routinely re-examined after a month. A tumour which has persisted or grown at that examination is an indication for laparotomy.

Multiple lutein cysts are associated with trophoblastic disease.

Corpus luteal cysts present with menstrual irregularities. The disordered sex hormone production with high androstenedione levels which accompanies **polycystic ovarian disease** is reflected in the secondary amenorrhoea, hirsutism, obesity, and infertility which are characteristic of this condition. The ovaries are bilaterally enlarged. **Benign ovarian fibromata** may present with ascites and a pleural effusion (Meig's syndrome), although most present as an incidental finding or with torsion where they are pedunculated. Some of the **tumours of the stroma** are associated with hormone production. The granulosa and theca cell tumours produce oestrogens and present with menstrual irregularities (see Chapter 2); the androblastoma secretes androgens, which lead to amenorrhoea and masculinization of the secondary sexual characteristics.

Neoplastic ovarian growths derive from the epithelium, germ cells, or gonadal stroma. The commonest large ovarian tumour is the **mucinous cystadenoma** derived from the epithelium, which can achieve massive proportions. Large cysts may be accompanied by wasting symptoms suggestive of malignancy. The cystadenoma contains multiple mucin-filled cysts separated by thin walls of fibrous tissue and columnar epithelium. Rupture of such a cyst may lead to seedling growths on the peritoneal surface.

Serous papilliferous growths also derive from the epithelium. The malignant variety is the commonest malignant ovarian neoplasm, and 50 per cent are bilateral. The tumour penetrates the cyst capsule and gives rise to multiple peritoneal seedling metastases, which spread rapidly in most cases.

The **dermoid cyst** is the commonest germ-cell tumour, having a peak incidence in the third decade of life. It is thought to arise from the division of unfertilized oocytes, and 20 per cent are bilateral. It consists of a single cyst with a mass at one end containing elements of differentiated tissues, such as skin, hair, teeth, and glandular and nervous tissue. Thyroid hormones may be secreted.

The most common malignant germ-cell tumour is the **dysgerminoma**, which is a highly malignant tumour of the second and third decades of life. There is an association with testicular feminization.

Ovarian cancer spreads by local infiltration, peritoneal seeding, lymphatic spread, and, rarely, blood-borne metastases. Ultrasonography is the investigation of choice.

Torsion of an ovarian or para-ovarian mass, pedunculated uterine fibromyoma, or normal adnexa presents with severe acute iliac fossa pain, which may radiate to the loin or groin.

Torsion is particularly characteristic of dermoid cysts and fibromata. There may be a history of previous episodes of similar pain, and the pain itself is often intermittent and colicky in nature. Nausea and vomiting may be present. Slight blood loss *per vaginam* may occur. There may be intra-peritoneal haemorrhage. A tender mass may be palpable. There may be a mild anaemia and a raised white-cell count.

Rupture of an ovarian or endometriotic cyst characteristically presents with sudden, constant pain that slowly subsides. If the cyst is large there may be severe pain, with vomiting and hypotension. On examination there is tenderness in the lateral and posterior fornices; a residual mass may occasionally be felt, and there may be peritonism or frank peritonitis.

Ultrasonography and/or laparoscopy may assist in the differential diagnosis of rupture from torsion. Urgent laparotomy is indicated where torsion has occurred. **Haemorrhage** into a cyst may occur, giving a clinical picture very like that of torsion.

Rarely a cyst may become **infected** after abortion or delivery or in association with the inflammation of another pelvic structure (for example in appendicitis).

Apart from the painful complications of torsion, rupture, and haemorrhage depicted above, *malignant and endometriotic tumours* may present with pain *a priori*. Severe pain is a common feature of germ-cell tumours.

Uterine perforation may follow IUCD insertion or currettage. It may also be the presenting feature of uterine carcinoma.

Characteristically, it presents with a dull ache, which intensifies as bleeding continues. Most bleeds are self-limiting; but laparotomy may be indicated.

The pain of the acute episode of **pelvic inflammatory disease** is characteristically bilateral, throbbing, and confined to the lower abdomen. Examination reveals a purulent vaginal discharge, marked tenderness in both fornices, and cervical excitation. If an abscess forms and ruptures the pain is severe, and gives rise to the signs first of localized, and then of generalized, peritonitis. Septic shock may supervene.

Exogenous gonadotrophins used in the treatment of infertility may lead to **ovarian hyperstimulation**. The sudden multiplication and enlargement of the follicles gives the clinical picture of diffuse lower abdominal pain, and cystic ovarian enlargement on palpation. Ascites, hydrothorax, and vascular thrombosis may occur. The severely affected patient becomes hypotensive, with a *raised* haematocrit.

If cervical or uterine carcinoma obstructs the internal os, entrapment and subsequent infection of the uterine contents ensues, causing a **pyometra**. The patient presents with uterine contractions, discharge, and slight enlargement of the uterus on vaginal examination. Ultrasound confirms the condition, which is relieved by dilatation of the cervix.

Patients presenting with chronic pelvic pain

- **Differential diagnosis of chronic pelvic pain**

The approach to the differential diagnosis of chronic pelvic pain is summarized in Box 3.2.

Pelvic pain may also be a manifestation of systemic disease, for example sickle cell, SLE.

Pain related to the menstrual cycle

The distinction between **dysmenorrhoea** that is caused by pelvic disease and the so-called 'primary' manifestation may be difficult. Both are felt in the lower abdomen and back, and both ache and may be colicky in nature. That associated with disease may start days, rather than hours before the period (endometriosis, salpingo-oophoritis); there may be associated symptoms such as menorrhagia; and the pain may represent a change, coming on after years of relatively pain-free menses. 'Primary' dysmenorrhoea occurs on the first day or two of the period, is a complaint of the late teens and early twenties, and is usually held by the patient to have always accompanied menstruation. The pathological basis is unclear, but a central role has been postulated for PGF2α. Treatment of the acute attack with analgesia and hot baths may be combined with prostaglandin inhibitors such as mefenamic acid. If pregnancy is not currently desired a progestogen, or combined progestogen–oestrogen, contraceptive pill is effective. The intra-uterine contraceptive device is not uncommonly associated with dysmenorrhoea and menorrhagia for the first couple of periods after insertion. Should dysmenorrhoea persist, a change of contraceptive method should be advised.

Premenstrual tension is a more common complaint in the third decade of life. The syndrome is characterized by a feeling of bloating days before the period, accompanied by weight gain, headache, irritability, depression, aggression, tearfulness, and impaired concentration and motivation. Patients may present to the emergency department com-

Box 3.2 **The differential diagnosis of chronic pelvic pain when pregnancy is not suspected**

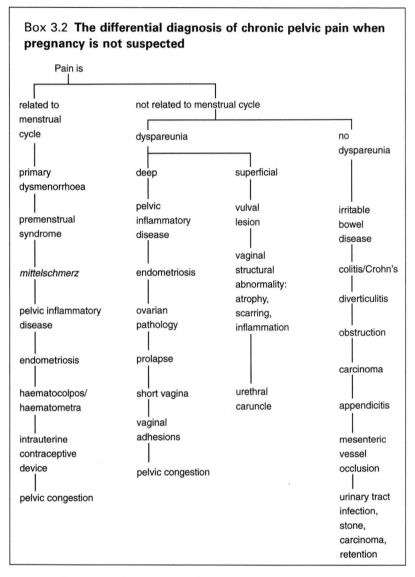

plaining of the psychological manifestations, or may be brought because of aggressive behaviour. Referral to both psychiatric and gynaecological services may need to be made. Norethisterone 5 mg twice a day in the latter half of the cycle, mild diuretics if weight gain is a marked feature, and low-dose diazepam may be useful holding measures whilst awaiting OPD evaluation.

Mittelschmerz is the name given to the mid-cycle iliac fossa pain which accompanies ovulation in some women. It is caused by the intraperitoneal extravasation of blood from the ovulating follicle. Sufferers are usually aged below thirty. The pain may last from minutes to two days, is usually mild but may be severe, may be referred to the shoulder-tip, and rarely may even be accompanied by syncope. There may be mid-cycle bleeding.

Both **endometriosis** and **pelvic inflammatory disease** present with constant lower abdominal pain and backache which worsen pre-menstrually. Tender enlarged adnexae may be found in both conditions, and laparoscopy will be needed to make the definitive diagnosis.

An imperforate hymen, or vaginal atresia, lead to the presentation of the patient with the rare condition of **haematocolpos**. The patient presents with the appearances of puberty, cyclical lower abdominal cramping pain and apparent primary amenorrhoea. Urinary retention may ensue. The vaginal abnormality and a pelvic mass are evident on examination.

A **haematometra,** blood trapped in the uterine cavity, may accompany a haematocolpos or may present as secondary amenorrhoea and cyclical pain. It is caused by iatrogenic stenosis of the cervix or by carcinoma occluding the internal os. Uterine abnormalities, such as a rudimentary horn or double uterus, may present with a haematometra that is disguised by normal menstruation from the remaining uterus.

Pelvic varicosities may cause the syndrome of **pelvic congestion**, which leads to complaints of cyclic dyspareunia, dysmenorrhoea, and abdominal tenderness in the multiparous patient. The pain is exacerbated by movement, and is usually unilateral.

Dyspareunia

Where unilateral oophorectomy and hysterectomy have been performed, the **residual ovary** may enlarge into a cystic tender mass which gives rise to chronic lower abdominal pain, sometimes accompanied by dyspareunia. An **ovarian remnant** remaining after bilateral salpingo-oophorectomy may present with dyspareunia and pelvic pain.

Uterine and vaginal wall **prolapse** are accompanied by a heavy feeling in the pelvis and backache which are relieved by lying down. Deep dyspareunia also results from **retroversion** of the uterus, and a **narrow or short vagina**. Tethering of the uterus to the pelvic structures by **adhesions** may also be culpable.

Vulval dystrophies or carcinoma present with local symptoms, including superficial dyspareunia.

Primary atrophy is characteristically noted around the time of the menopause; but atrophy may occur without the menopause and vice versa. The skin is red and shiny, the labia minora lose bulk, and the introitus shrinks. Surrounding skin is not affected. The condition can progress to leukoplakia and malignancy.

The irregularly hypertrophied whitened areas of **hypoplastic and hyperplastic vulval dystrophy** affect the inner labia majora, labia minora, introitus, and prepuce. The soreness and dyspareunia associated with these conditions may respond to dienoestrol cream or oral oestrogens. Long-term follow-up is mandatory, as they are sometimes premalignant.

Vulval squamous cell carcinoma may be found. The disease is more common in elderly women, and is associated with dystrophic changes in the vulva in the majority of cases. Vulval dystrophy, lymphogranuloma inguinale, granuloma venereum, and schistosomiasis are predisposing factors. Lymphatic spread is early, bleeding may occur, and infection supervenes to cause an offensive discharge. Local erosion may lead to haemorrhage from the femoral vessels. Treatment is surgical, with irradiation of recurrences.

Bartholin's abscesses form by infection of the cystic enlargement of a blocked Bartholin's duct. They present as a painful swelling on the inner side of the posterior end of the labium majus. Treatment is by admission for surgery.

Primary *Herpes simplex* is extremely painful. There may be a history of infection in the partner. On examination shallow ulcers with a yellowish base and bright red edges are seen on the vulva and may be found in the vagina, on the cervix, and around the perineal area or lower abdomen. Vaginal speculum examination is often impossible as it is so painful. Vaginal swabs may be taken without the speculum, for viral studies and also for bacterial culture for concurrent infection. If the patient is not pregnant, acyclovir topically or orally is helpful.

Secondary *Herpes simplex* infection of the vulva, perineal area, or buttock lasts about a week, with a history of previous similar episodes at the same site. Acyclovir cream or tablets may reduce the length of the attack.

If the patient is pregnant acyclovir is contraindicated. The pregnant patient must be told to inform her obstetrician of the infection and to report immediately to hospital if her membranes rupture. Caesarean section may be needed to prevent infection of the fetus.

Behçet's syndrome may cause shallow painful ulcers on the vulva. Systemic manifestations, such as arthralgia and iritis, aid the diagnosis.

The indolent, deep, large, **ulcers of Lipshutz** may be the source of severe vulval pain.

Malignant melanoma and basal-cell carcinoma may also affect the vulva.

Lesions of the urethral meatus and vaginal structural abnormalities (for example an intact hymen or vaginal septum) or inflammation may also present with superficial dyspareunia.

Further reading

Rocker, L. (ed.) (1990). *Diagnosis and management of pelvic pain in women.* Springer-Verlag, Berlin.

Salat-Baroux, J. and Antoine, J. M. (1990). Accidental hyperstimulation during ovulation induction. *Baillière's Clinical Obstetrics and Gynaecology,* **4** (3), 627–37.

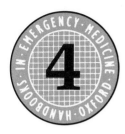

CHAPTER 4

The patient presenting with vaginal discharge

Key points on the patient presenting with vaginal discharge

1 Patients presenting with infective vaginitis, cervicitis, and pelvic inflammatory disease *must* have follow-up arranged in the genito-urinary or gynaecology out-patient clinic.

2 Patients who present with atrophic vaginitis accompanied by a discharge through the cervical os, must not be commenced on oestrogen therapy until uterine carcinoma has been ruled out.

Differential diagnosis of discharge *per vaginam*

An approach to the differential diagnosis of discharge *per vaginam* is outlined in Box 4.1.

If no local inflammation or abnormality is found on examination, the apparent increase in discharge may be physiological, or there may be anaerobic vaginosis (for example, from *Gardnerella vaginalis*).

Gardnerella vaginalis gives rise to a greyish, bubbly, offensive discharge unaccompanied by vaginitis. Wet slides show 'clue' cells, epithelial cells with a speckled appearance due to bacteria fixed to their surface. The organism can be cultured from a sample taken into Stuart's transport medium. The infection is treated with metronidazole 400 mg twice a day for 7 days.

Vaginitis

The vast majority of cases of **infective vaginitis** are caused by ***Candida albicans*** or ***Trichomonas vaginalis***. Both infections are common in pregnancy. Diabetes, the contraceptive pill, and antibiotics also pre-dispose to candidal infection. Trichomonal infection is usually sexually transmitted, but cross-infection (for example from toilet articles, or instruments in gynaecological clinics) may occur. On examination the vaginal wall is reddened and congested, and there may be accompanying vulvitis. Minute punctate ulceration of the vaginal wall may be seen in trichomonal infection. The discharge is characteristically thick and white with candidal infection, and profuse, thin, yellow, and offensive with trichomonal infection. Wet preparations will show the mycelial threads of *Candida albicans* or the protozoon of *Trichomonas vaginalis*. Both organisms may be cultured from swabs; ideally that for *Trichomonas* should be placed in specialist transport medium.

Suspected candidal infection is conveniently treated with

Box 4.1 **An approach to the diagnosis of vaginal discharge**

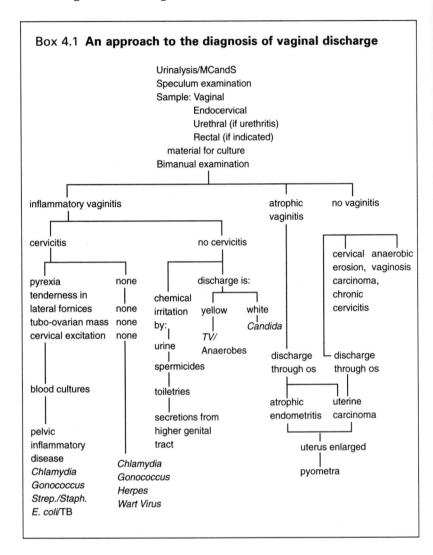

a single-dose clotrimazole 500 mg pessary. Suspected trichomonal infection is treated with metronidazole 400 mg twice
a day for one week, prescribed to both partners, who must
abstain from alcohol during the treatment. Patients with
infective vaginitis must be followed up in the genito-urinary

medicine clinic. Either organism may infect the sexual partner, and other infections may be evident on the results of the laboratory cultures, *Trichomonas* in particular being associated with gonococcal infection.

Women may present to the emergency department complaining of **chemical vaginitis** due to the leakage of urine or faeces *per vaginam*. Vesicovaginal, ureterovaginal, and rectovaginal fistulae may result from obstetric or peroperative injury, from sexual abuse, or from neoplastic invasion. Colovaginal fistulae may complicate acute diverticulitis. Where there is leakage of urine the anterior vaginal wall should be inspected with a Sims' speculum.

In this country, most fistulae between the urinary and genital tracts are caused by peroperative injury, are small, and are located high on the anterior vaginal wall. Patients from countries with poor obstetric services may present with large fistulae in the middle of the vaginal wall caused by necrosis secondary to prolonged labour. Rectovaginal fistulae usually follow third-degree tears of the perineum which are unrepaired, or the repair of which has broken down. Referral (usually as an outpatient) to the gynaecologist for operative repair is indicated in all cases.

Chemical vaginitis may also result from irritation by spermicides, toiletries and secretions from higher genital tract pathology.

Atrophic vaginitis begins as oestrogen levels drop after the menopause. The vaginal and vulval epithelium thins, there is a fall in glycogen levels in the epithelial cells, and the vaginal pH rises. There is a profuse, yellow, sometimes bloodstained discharge. Examination shows redness and shininess of the vulva and inflammation of the rather smooth vaginal wall, and adhesions may form in the vagina. Treatment is by local or systemic oestrogens.

Cervicitis

Acute cervicitis rarely exists as an isolated abnormality, usually being associated with a generalized genital tract infection. The cervix is red and congested, with a purulent exudate. Herpes (see Chapter 3) and wart viruses, Chlamydia, and Gonococcus may be responsible, and the condition may follow dilatation, abortion, or childbirth. Mild urethritis, infection of Bartholin's glands, and (rarely) iritis, arthritis, and endocarditis may accompany gonococcal cervicitis. Chlamydial infection responds to a fortnight's course of oxytetracycline 500 mg four times a day, or erythromycin 500 mg twice a day where tetracyclines are contraindicated. Gonococcal infection may be treated with ampicillin 3 g, with probenecid 1 g or cefotaxime 1 g intramuscularly. Referral to a genito-urinary medicine clinic is mandatory.

Chronic cervicitis gives rise to a mucopurulent discharge, often accompanied by pelvic pain, backache, and dyspareunia. The cervix contains multiple nabothian follicles (cervical gland retention cysts). Most cases develop after bacterial infection during abortion, instrumentation, or childbirth; some may be caused by Chlamydia or tuberculosis.

Pelvic inflammatory disease

Pelvic inflammatory disease is a blanket term used to cover endometritis, salpingitis, oophoritis, parametritis, and local peritoneal or bowel involvement. The majority of cases are chlamydial. Gonococci, streptococci, staphylococci, coliforms, actinomycosis, and tuberculosis may be found. Most infection ascends from the lower genital tract, but some cases arise from the local spread of infection from the gut or pelvic peritoneum or from blood-borne infection. In the **acute** condition, the fallopian tubes become inflamed and oedematous, with epithelial damage and a purulent exudate; adhesions form within the tube, trapping the exudate to cause a pyosalpinx; and inflammation may spread through the wall of the tube, causing local peritoneal irritation and adhesions between the tube and other pelvic structures. The leakage of infected exudate from the fimbrial end of the tube may give rise to pelvic peritonitis and abscesses and to involvement of the ovaries, which become swollen, and in which small abscesses may form. The patient is unwell, in pain, pyrexial, and tachycardic, with a vaginal discharge, peritonism over both iliac fossae, marked lateral forniceal tenderness, and cervical excitation. Vomiting may occur early, and rigors may accompany abscess formation. Menstrual irregularities are common. There may be a general feeling of fullness in the lateral fornices, or a frank pelvic mass may be palpable. A peritubal abscess may drain into the rectum. The clinical picture resembles appendicitis. Some aids to the differential diagnosis are given in Box 4.2. Laparoscopic examination will give the definitive diagnosis.

Box 4.2 **The differential diagnosis of PID and appendicitis**

Pelvic inflammatory disease	Appendicitis
Sexually active, known STD risk, recent abortion or delivery	Not necessarily
Pain bilateral, lower abdominal	Pain periumbilical, then right iliac fossa
High pyrexia	Pyrexia rarely exceeds 38.5°
Vomiting early and inconstant	Vomiting common
Both fornices tender	Usually right only

Treatment may be given as an outpatient, although severe cases should be admitted for intravenous therapy. Bedrest, fluids, and analgesia should be combined with an initial dose of 1.5 g cefuroxime followed by a two-week course of oxytetracycline 500 mg four times a day and metronidazole 400 mg three times a day. Where tetracycline is contraindicated (for example in pregnancy) erythromycin 500 mg four times a day may be used. Where an IUCD is present this should be removed once antibiotic cover is established, and sent for culture. The patient should be referred for gynaecological/genito-urinary medicine follow-up; in the meantime sexual abstinence should be advised until the patient's partner has been evaluated and treated.

The **chronic** form may follow an acute episode; or the initial infection may have been clinically mild and have gone unrecognized. Irregular menstruation, with dysmenorrhoea, dyspareunia, dull lower abdominal pain and backache, general malaise with fatigue, and a low pyrexia are common. On examination there may be a discharge, the tubes are thickened and tender, and cervical excitation may be noted. Antibiotic treatment will be needed for up to six months, and surgery may be the only curative measure.

Infertility and ectopic pregnancy may result from acute or chronic infection. Ophthalmia neonatorum and neonatal pneumonia may develop in babies born to mothers with chlamydial infection, and conjunctivitis in those born to mothers with gonococcal infection.

Endometritis

When the patient with atrophic vaginitis is examined, a discharge may be seen passing through the internal os; this may be due to accompanying **atrophic endometritis**, but the possibility of uterine carcinoma must be borne in mind. Post-menopause the rise in vaginal pH, diminution in cervical mucus, and cessation of periodic shedding of the endometrium allow infection to ascend into the endometrium. There is a purulent, bloodstained discharge, and a pyometra may supervene, giving tender enlargement of the uterus. The patient should be referred for gynaecological assessment before treatment. Dilatation and curettage to facilitate drainage and exclude carcinoma are performed, systemic oestrogen is given, and rapid healing is to be expected. Recurrence is rare.

Primary syphilis

Primary syphilis may present with a serous or purulent discharge from the primary chancre, which is usually located on the cervix, but may be found on the labia. On examination there is a non-tender, shallow ulcer with well-defined edges and a smooth floor. The labia may be generally swollen, and there may be local painless lymphadenopathy. Secondary bacterial infection may supervene. Referral to a department of genito-urinary medicine must be made. Diagnosis is by the finding of spirochaetes on dark-ground microscopy, and treatment by intramuscular procaine penicillin.

Further reading

Kahn, J. G., Walker, C. K., Washington, A. E., Landers, D. V., and Sweet, R. L. (1991). Diagnosing Pelvic Inflammatory Disease, a comprehensive analysis and considerations for developing a new model. *Journal of the American Medical Association*, **266** (18), 2594–604.

Roberts, D. and McCullough, A. (1990). Infections of the vulva and vagina. In *Clinical infections in obstetrics and gynaecology* (ed. A. B. Maclean), pp. 262–73. Blackwell Scientific Publications, Oxford.

Sobel, J. D. (1990). Bacterial vaginosis. *British Journal of Clinical Practice*, **71**, 65–9.

Stacey, C. M., Barton, S. E., and Singer, A. (1991). In *Progress in obstetrics and gynaecology*, Vol. 9 (ed. J. Studd), pp. 259–71. Churchill Livingstone, Edinburgh.

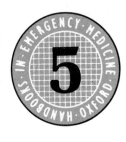

CHAPTER 5

The patient presenting with genital injury or assault

Key points in the patient presenting with genital injury or assault

1 Abdominal injury in the pregnant patient may be the presenting picture of domestic violence.

2 The incidence of domestic violence is grossly underestimated in A and E practice, and the consequences of the lack of identification of the problem are potentially grave. Crisis intervention is imperative.

3 Rape victims may be too emotionally traumatized to wish to report the crime at the time they present to A and E. The emergency physician should collect and preserve, or arrange for the collection and preservation of, forensic evidence in case the victim subsequently decides to pursue a prosecution.

4 The records of injuries and other evidence of assault must be meticulously completed, with photographs, notes, and specimens, timed, dated, and signed.

5 Rape victims should be offered post-coital contraception where there is a risk of pregnancy, and follow-up in the genito-urinary clinic must be arranged.

6 Victims of violence need on-going psychological and practical support. Agencies are listed in the text of this chapter and in Appendix 1.

Blunt trauma

The usual mechanism of blunt injury to the vulva or vagina is a straddle injury. Aggressive sexual activity or sexual assault may also cause perineal injury. Most vulval haematomata will settle with ice-packs and time; however, evacuation under anaesthesia will be needed if the haematoma is large. Vaginal lacerations from rape or foreign-body insertion are best explored and repaired under general anaesthesia. Forgotten tampons and other foreign bodies may cause local ulceration.

Penetrating trauma

Intrauterine contraceptive devices may migrate through the myometrium. Uterine perforation may follow IUCD sounding or insertion especially if it is sited post-partum. IUCD migration or perforation may present with increasing pain from peritoneal irritation, with peritonitis, bowel obstruction, cystitis, rectal or vaginal bleeding, and pregnancy; or may be asymptomatic. Signs include disappearance of the IUCD string and breaking of the string during attempts to dislodge the IUCD. The IUCD may be located by ultrasound or X-ray. A small perforation may heal without incident; others cause a haemoperitoneum and require laparotomy. If the IUCD itself is judged to have penetrated the uterine wall, laparotomy is mandatory.

Perforation may also accompany intra-uterine instrumentation during termination of pregnancy, or diagnostic curettage. The resultant pain may be immediate or delayed, depending on the course of intraperitoneal bleeding and infection. Any patient with significant blood loss or infection requires immediate laparotomy. Perforations by blunt instruments may be watched in hospital; penetrations by sharp instruments require operative exclusion of damage to other pelvic structures.

Domestic violence

Pregnancy is a recognized precipitant of violence in the home: 13 per cent of victims of partner abuse suffer their first assault whilst pregnant, and the severity of pre-existing domestic violence worsens in 30 per cent of cases when the woman becomes pregnant. Abdominal injury in the pregnant patient may, therefore, be the presenting episode. Rape and genital injury are commonly seen in partner abuse.

Sadly, domestic violence often goes unsuspected and unremarked upon in the emergency department, where the care team have a unique chance to support the victim and, if invited, to intervene. As the psychological state and social situation of the abused woman make her a poor keeper of follow-up appointments, crisis intervention is imperative. A brief outline of the problem is therefore given in Boxes 5.1, 5.2, 5.3, 5.4 and 5.5.

Box 5.1 **Presentation of the female victim of domestic violence**

A. History
Domestic violence affects women of all classes, races, and creeds.

Presenting complaints	Pattern of attendance
Injury, often multiple	Patient attends late
Rape	Partner answers for patient
Suicide/parasuicide	Over-vehement denial of
Psychiatric illness/	abuse
substance abuse	May be frequent attender
Pelvic pain	On multiple prescribed
Multiple somatic	drugs
complaints	Patient not rarely pregnant

Box 5.2 **Presentation of the female victim of domestic violence**

B. Examination

Indicators of abuse	Characteristic injuries
Patient is:	Facial injury
evasive	Perforated eardrums
embarrassed/apologetic	Detached retina
anxious/depressed	Neck injury, esp. marks
passive	Breast injury
	To abdomen when
Injuries:	pregnant
affect areas normally	Genital injury
covered	Burns/scalds
inconsistent with	Bruises
mechanism stated	Bizarre injuries
at multiple sites	
symmetrically	
distributed	

Box 5.3 **Presentation of the female victim of domestic violence**

C. Documentation
Document meticulously; photograph injuries with patient's written consent. Sign and date all notes and photographs, and attach firmly to patient's medical record.

Record:
Time, date, place of abuse
Witnesses to incident
Injury size, pattern, age, location
Signs of sexual abuse
Non-bodily evidence, for example torn clothing
Patient's explanation
Your opinion *re* causation

Box 5.4 **Approach to the victim of domestic violence**

Maintain a high level of suspicion.
Exclude partner, interview in privacy, stress confidentiality.

- Ask direct questions gently, stating that domestic violence is common and it is routine to enquire about home circumstances where there is a possibility of abuse on clinical grounds.
- Be non-judgemental: do not directly condemn partner; do not criticize patient for staying with him.
- Emphasize the appropriateness of the patient's attendance.
- Focus on informing the patient: stress that violence in the home is illegal, that expert help is available, and that legal intervention is possible. Supply contact details for support organizations, for example Women's Aid.
- Discuss safety: How much at risk does the patient feel—of homicide?—of suicide? Are there weapons in the house? What has she tried before? What sources of support does she have? What possible safe havens? Are there children? Are they safe? Help her examine her options.
- Move at the patient's own pace. Nurture the patient's right to make her own decisions.

Rape

Rape is penetration of the vulva or beyond by the male genitalia without the consent of the woman, or when the woman lacks the ability to consent owing to physical or mental incapacity (including intoxication). Both the real incidence of rape and the frequency of reporting of this act of violence are rising, and estimates place the level of risk of rape or attempted rape at one in five women. Police planning is making increasing provision for this crime, and there are

Box 5.5 **Treatment of the victim of domestic violence**

- Treat the physical illness or injury
- Seek psychiatric help where depression is prominent or for parasuicide.
- Hospitalize 'for social reasons' if there is no other safe option, or the patient is too emotionally exhausted to make her own decisions.
- If the patient is returning to her partner: give her contact numbers and written information (on legal options, help available, etc.), offer referral, help her plan an escape route for emergencies, advise her to keep money and important financial and legal documents hidden in a safe place. If the children are at risk, consider referral to social services, preferably with the patient's consent.
- If the patient does not wish to return and needs a place of safety: consider friends or relatives, try emergency housing (contact duty social worker), contact local refuge; police may offer protected accommodation; hospitalize if all else fails.
- Domestic violence is a crime like any other, and prosecution for aggravated bodily harm, rape, etc. follows standard lines. The victim may also have recourse to the civil law (non-molestation, exclusion orders, etc.).
- Refer to Women's Aid, GP, social work, police, family planning, Rape Crisis, etc. as indicated and requested.

now rape suites and investigation teams throughout the country. The emergency physician must be similarly prepared with a well-developed protocol for management. This should include the provision of a quiet private area equipped for a pelvic examination, and agreements with police, social services, hospital and crime laboratories, and voluntary aid agencies about the role of each in the assessment and care of the victim. The emergency department staff should be trained in their approach to the victim, with emphasis on

5.6 Emergency team's approach to the rape victim

- Introduction of self
- Reassurance that the patient is safe
- Empathetic listening to the patient's ordeal
- Supportive informing of the patient of her physical condition
- Involvement of the patient in procedures and decision-making
- Brief discussion of the psychological sequelae of rape with the patient
- Arranging for supportive follow-up (which may include a safe haven)

the safety of the patient's surroundings, the return of the patient's right to consent or deny, and the expression of active support and concern. Written consent should be obtained whenever physically possible, both to the pelvic examination and to the release of evidence to the prosecuting authorities. Box 5.6 summarizes the basic approach.

Forensically, the physician's role has three elements: ensuring that evidence is not accidentally destroyed; working with the forensic medical examiner where the rape is reported to the police and the degree of injury requires the input of the hospital service; and taking on the role of the forensic medical service in collecting evidence when the crime is not reported, in case the victim subsequently decides to prosecute. The local forensic medical examiner may be willing to collect such evidence, even when the rape has not been reported to the police.

Both hospital and pre-hospital staff should be careful to disturb as little evidence at the site of the attack or on the victim as is commensurate with ensuring the patient's physical safety until formal collection of forensic material is possible. Box 5.7 outlines the points to be covered when taking a history of a rape, and Box 5.8 details the specimens required in evidence and the method of their preservation. The victim is asked to stand on a piece of paper whilst undressing, to catch debris which might be useful in evidence. If the patient is unconscious, the paper stretcher cover should be retained. If semen, blood, etc. has dried on to the skin swabs may be moistened with tap or sterile water (not normal saline). External and internal vaginal swabs must be taken for examination for saliva, semen, and lubricants. The internal vaginal swabs should be taken from both the low and the high vagina. When more than two days have elapsed since the rape, an endocervical swab should be substituted for the high vaginal swab. Documentation is all-important. Each stage of the assessment of the patient should be timed, and details of all personnel involved should be recorded. Each sample must be recorded and labelled with details of from whom and from where the sample came, when and by whom it

---

Box 5.7 **Points to cover when taking a history of rape**

● Day, date, time, and location of the assault
● Number of assailants
● Assailant's approach to victim
● Non-sexual assault, if any
● Removal of, or possible damage to, clothing
● Sexual assault: mouth, vagina, anus, breasts, skin
● Lubricant used
● Condom used
● Drugs/alcohol involved
● Actions afterwards
　　—changed clothes
　　—washed/bathed/showered
　　—urinated/defecated
　　—replaced tampon/sanitary towel
　　—mouth wash/gargle/cleaned teeth
　　—drinks/when taken
　　—medication/when taken
● Sexual intercourse since assault
● Sexual intercourse prior to assault (if within two weeks)
● Alcohol/drugs/medication taken immediately before assault
● Previous general medical, gynaecological, and obstetric history

was taken, and to whom and where it was passed. These details must include a reference number and sample description (for example Case X No. 1/Saliva; Case X No. 2/ Urine). The person packing, labelling, and sealing the sample must sign the label. Each stage of this process must be double-checked.

Victims are degraded by their experience, and may be too embarrassed to reveal the full details of the assault. Saliva samples should be routinely taken for examination for evidence of oral assault. Clues to anal assault include anal spasm on examination, difficulty in taking the anal swabs, and a complaint of pain on defecation. The latter persists for a few days after the assault.

About 1 per cent of rape victims become pregnant. If there

Box 5.8 **Forensic examination of the rape victim**

- Observe damage to, staining of, and materials adhering to clothing
- Full medical examination, charting of injuries
- Photographs of injuries if possible
- Take forensic samples, i.e.:

Sample	Placed in	Preserved in
Sheet of paper	Paper bag	Dry storage
Clothing	Paper bag	Dry storage
Blood group/DNA profile	EDTA	Fridge
Blood alcohol	Fluoride/Oxalate	Fridge
Saliva/sperm group	Glass/plastic bottle	Fridge
Urine drugs/alcohol	Sodium fluoride	Fridge
Loose alien hairs/debris	Plastic bag/tube	Dry storage
Fingernail clippings	Plastic bag	Dry storage
Skin swabs	Plastic tube	Freeze
Vaginal/cervical swabs	Plastic tube	Freeze
Tampon/sanitary towel	Plastic bag	Freeze
Anal swabs	Plastic bag	Freeze

is a risk of conception, a pre-existing pregnancy should first be excluded by βHCG testing, and then postcoital contraception may be offered. If this fails, or the patient presents late, referral for termination of pregnancy may be offered. About 3 per cent of rape victims develop sexually transmitted infections. Follow-up examination in a genitourinary diseases clinic must be arranged. The patient's reluctance to re-attend may be helped by being accompanied by the police officer concerned with her case or by a counsellor's support and advice. One regime is a consultation two days after the rape, to establish the previous relevant history and perform baseline tests, followed by another at three weeks. HIV testing may be requested or offered. As well as the baseline sample, an HIV test should be taken three months after the assault. The psychological impact of rape is considerable; long-term sequelae include post-traumatic stress disorder, anxiety states, phobias, and depression, as well as psychosexual difficulties. Follow-up from this perspective is indispensable, either by health service personnel or by volunteer counsellors (for example Rape Crisis).

The patient's physical well-being should also be checked either by the hospital or the patient's own doctor. Routine reassessment at two and six weeks has been suggested.

Female circumcision

Despite being illegal in most countries, this mutilation is still practised across sub-Saharan Africa, and in the western world by people from those countries. Circumcision is performed in infancy or at puberty, with the degree of trauma varying from removal of the tip of the clitoris and parts of the labia majora, to excision of the labia minora and clitoris and fusion of the vulva, leaving only a minute hole for urination. Early complications include local and systemic infection, haemorrhage, and urethral injury. First coitus may be traumatic, with further local damage, haemorrhage, and subsequent infection and scarring. Late complications include haematocolpos, pyocolpos, vaginal stenosis, and obstructed labour. Caesarean section is indicated where the mutilation is extensive or vaginal stenosis is severe.

Further reading

Eckert, W. G., Katchis, S., and Donovan, W. (1991). The pathology and medicolegal aspects of sexual activity. *American Journal of Forensic Medicine and Pathology*, **12** (1), 3–15.

Glaser, J. B., Hammerschlag, M. R., and McCormack, W. M. (1989). Epidemiology of sexually transmitted disease in rape victims. *Reviews of Infectious Diseases*, **11** (2), 246–54.

Home Office (1989). *Domestic violence*, Home Office Research Study 107. HMSO, London.

Lightfoot-Klein, H. and Shaw, E. (1991). Special needs of ritually circumcised women patients. *Journal of Obstetrics, Gynaecologic and Neonatal Nursing*, **20** (2), 102–7.

Victim Support (1992). *Domestic violence. Report of a multidisciplinary working party.* Victim Support, London.

CHAPTER 6

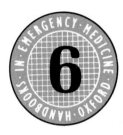

Gynaecology in childhood and adolescence

Key points in gynaecology in childhood and adolescence

1 Whenever possible, the number of intimate examinations of the child or adolescent should be limited by the immediate involvement of the paediatric and gynaecological specialist teams.

2 The possibility of sexual abuse must always be borne in mind. Where it is suspected, the child abuse team must be immediately called.

3 Emergency department examination of the pre-menarchal child should be limited to inspection of the external genitalia.

4 The possibility of pregnancy must be remembered when assessing the post-menarchal child.

Techniques of pelvic examination in children

The approach to the **gynaecological assessment** of a child must be gentle and sympathetic. For most children the genital examination will be the first of its type. The number of examinations necessary should be limited where possible by the immediate involvement of paediatric and/or gynaecological specialists. Where sexual abuse or assault is suspected, it is even more important that every effort should be made to minimize the psychological trauma to the child, and assessments are best conducted by the local child-abuse team, although the facilities and skills of the A and E department may be needed for accompanying physical trauma. Each examination must commence with an explanation of the procedure to the child and reassurance that it is not painful.

In all post-pubertal adolescents the possibility of pregnancy must be borne in mind, and the comments on abortion, ectopia, etc. made in the other chapters of this book apply.

The examination commences with the usual general examination, including the lymph glands and fauces, and the Tanner stage (Table 6.1).

In the **premenarchal child**, pelvic examination should be

Table 6.1 • Tanner staging of puberty

Stage	Pubic hair	Breast development
1	None	Elevation of papilla only
2	Sparse, on labia majora only	Breast budding, areolar enlargement, and mound-like elevation of breast and papilla
3	Course, curly hair distributed sparsely over mons	Continued enlargement of breast and areola without separation of contours
4	Adult in character but not in distribution	Areola and papilla project above breast contour
5	Adult distribution, with spread to the inner thighs	Adult appearance, with areola recessed to breast contour

limited to inspection of the external genitalia. If internal examination is indicated by the presence of trauma or the suspicion of a foreign body, this should be performed under general anaesthesia. To examine the genitalia, the child may be held on the mother's lap supine in the 'frog's legs position'. The older child may take up the knee–chest position in Fig 6.1. An assistant then lifts the buttocks up and separates them, giving a view of the open vagina.

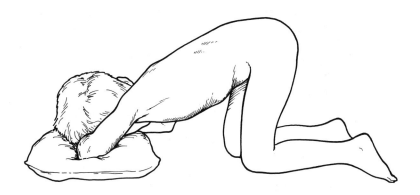

Fig. 6.1 • The 'Knees–chest' position.

Post-inflammatory labial adhesions may be evident on inspection of the young child; these should not be forcibly pulled apart.

Box 6.1 lists the expected hymenal opening size by age.

Box 6.1 **Hymenal opening by age**

Age	Hymenal opening (cm)
Less than two months	0.4
Two months to seven years	0.5
Seven to ten years	0.7
Ten years	1.0

The vagina should be inspected with magnification and a pen-torch. Instruments must not be used. Bimanual recto-abdominal examination (using the fifth finger in young children) may be used where nothing can be seen vaginally and a foreign body is suspected. Ultrasound examination is very valuable in this age-group, and may obviate the need for a distressing degree of exposure. Specimens for culture should be taken of any abnormal discharge.

Vaginal examination may be indicated by trauma, suspected abuse, discharge, bleeding, or pain in the **postmenarchal adolescent**. The same examination positions may be used as for adult women.

Sexually active patients, or those who have been using tampons routinely for menstruation, may be examined using a small Cusco or Sims' speculum. A cervical smear should be taken, and swabs for culture may be taken as routine. Where the hymenal opening is large bimanual examination may be performed as for the older patient. When vaginal examination is refused, a rectal examination may again prove informative.

Other patients are best examined under anaesthesia by the gynaecologist.

Precocious puberty

The first sign of puberty usually appears after the age of 9, and is enlargement of the breast buds, followed by pubic hair and accelerated growth and then the menarche at 11 years old onwards. **Precocious puberty** may be defined as the onset of puberty at less than 9 years old. Cases have been recorded as young as 4 years old. Alarmed parents may bring children to the emergency department. Most cases of precocious puberty have no sinister underlying cause, result only in mild growth retardation, and may be treated with gonadotrophin-releasing hormone analogues. However, granulosa cell tumours of the ovary, malignant teratomas, and, rarely, encephalitis, hydrocephalus, and lesions in the area of the hypothalamus, pituitary, pineal, and third ventricle, may present with breast and pubic hair growth and menstruation. Adrenal tumours may cause enlargement of the genitalia, but not uterine bleeding. The child should be referred as an outpatient to the paediatric department for further assessment.

Bleeding

Bleeding *per vaginam* may occur in the first ten days of life as a physiological response to hormonal changes. In the young child a foreign body should be sought. A small withdrawal bleed is not uncommon after a child has helped herself to the mother's contraceptive pill. Vaginal tumours may present in this age-group. **The possibility of sexual abuse or assault must always be considered.**

In the adolescent irregular bleeding may result from abortion, ectopia, vulvovaginitis, vaginal or cervical tumour, cervical erosion, salpingitis, and endometritis, as in the adult woman. Bleeding diatheses may cause excessive menstrual loss, as may IUCD use. Thyroid and adrenal disease may also be associated with menstrual irregularity. Dysfunctional uterine bleeding is common around the menarche when the menstrual cycles are anovulatory; nearly all cases recover spontaneously. The patient should be resuscitated as necessary and referred to paediatric and gynaecological teams.

Pelvic pain

Pelvic pain around puberty may be due to psychological, gastrointestinal, urinary, or gynaecological causes. A more valuable history may be taken with the parents excluded. The classic pattern of school phobia is of a pain which occurs during term-time and is better at the weekend. Psychogenic pain may also be an indicator of anxiety or depression, family pathology, and/or abuse. The complaint may be of dysmenorrhoea or *Mittelschmerz*, or an ovarian mass may be found on examination. Such masses may rupture or tort, and present with acute, severe pain. The highly malignant dysgerminoma is found in this age-group.

Where the girl is **sexually active**, pelvic inflammatory disease, ectopic pregnancy, and abortion should be considered and managed as for the mature woman.

The usual watchpoints of excluding pregnancy in all sexually active females complaining of abdominal pain, and of carefully examining for, and vigorously correcting, hypovolaemia apply.

Where there has been **no sexual activity** the pain may be caused by a **haematocolpos** caused by vaginal atresia. The obstruction is usually a membrane across the vagina located above the hymen. In some cases a segment, or the whole, of the vagina is absent. The rest of the genital tract is usually normal. Once menstruation starts, fluid slowly accumulates behind the membrane, some being reabsorbed between menses. The patient presents around the age of 15 with pain which may be severe. A history of monthly abdominal discomfort, apparent amenorrhoea, and developed secondary characteristics should suggest the diagnosis. Retention of urine and constipation may accompany the mass. On examination there is a lower abdominal mass, and a bulging membrane is visible on vulval inspection. Where the atresia is higher in the vagina, there may be no mass palpable and no membrane immediately visible. The patient should be referred immediately to the gynaecologists for excision of the membrane, under antibiotic cover and full operating theatre asepsis. Retrograde menstruation can result in endometriosis and in infertility due to adhesions of the fimbrial ends of the fallopian tubes. A similar condition may affect the newborn owing to the accumulation of cervical secretions behind the membrane.

Discharge

Discharge is usually due to physiological leucorrhoea. Newborn girls and those approaching puberty commonly have excess vaginal secretions. **The possibility of sexual abuse must be considered whenever a child presents with vaginal discharge.**

Once the first fortnight is past, discharge in the **neonate** may be due to congenital abnormalities of the genitourinary system which lead to the drainage of urine through the vagina or to the colonization of the vagina at birth with *Chlamydia*. The latter may persist for up to two years. Vulvovaginitis in the **premenarchal** child is usually due to poor hygiene. The parents and child should be advised on the use of daily washing, cotton undergarments, and 'simple' toiletries and washing powders, and the avoidance of deodorants and tampons. Skin conditions such as psoriasis or scabies may be seen on vulval examination. Chickenpox, measles, Stevens–Johnson syndrome, and inflammatory bowel disease may all be accompanied by vulvovaginitis. Streptococci, staphylococci, *H. influenzae*, *N. meningitidis*, and *Shigella* may cause vaginal infection, as well as the sexually transmitted diseases and *Candida*.

If there is itching which worsens at night the vaginitis may be caused by threadworms. Mebendazole 100 mg single dose may be used in children over two years old; piperazine 50–75 mg/kg once daily for seven days is recommended for children under two. Purulent or bloodstained discharge should raise the question of a foreign body, which may be removed with forceps or a saline flush; occasionally general anaesthesia is required.

Sexually active or abused children are affected by the same spectrum of infection as the adult.

Trauma

Lacerations of the vulva or perineum may be caused by falling on a sharp object, for instance a toy or a bicycle handlebar. The labia majora are the most common sites of injury. The wound is usually relatively trivial, but bleeding may be profuse if the laceration has penetrated deep to the labia. The bleeding should be controlled with direct pressure, the patient should be resuscitated as necessary, and referral should be made for exploration and repair under general anaesthesia if there is suspicion of deep penetration or the wound is of significant size or depth.

Blunt trauma, for example from falling astride a climbing frame, may result in **vulval or perineal haematomata**. The scale of the bleeding should be carefully assessed; the child should be asked to pass urine; and pelvic X-rays should be taken if the history merits it. Ice may be applied locally, and analgesia should be given as a routine. A pressure dressing may then be applied. If the haematoma is large or increasing in size, the child should be admitted for operative drainage and haemostasis. **Vaginal lacerations or haematoma** may also result from accidental injury or from foreign-body insertion by the child, but a particularly high suspicion of abuse must be maintained. If there is hymenal laceration, a vaginal examination is mandatory. Retroperitoneal bleeding from torn pelvic vessels may accompany vaginal trauma. Referral should be made to the gynaecology and paediatric teams for assessment and repair of lacerations, evacuation of haematomata (if necessary), and treatment of any associated injury under anaesthesia. The integrity of urethra, bladder, and bowel should be checked under the same anaesthetic. If the vaginal vault is lacerated, exploration of the pelvic cavity is indicated.

Sexual abuse

Sexual abuse is the most frequent form of child abuse: 25 per cent of girls and 10 per cent of boys are estimated to have been subjected to such abuse by the time they reach 18 years old. Most abusers are male adult members of the child's own household, although abuse by an adolescent brother is not rare. Box 6.2 outlines the characteristics of the family situation.

Direct indicators of abuse include recurrent vulvo-vaginitis, perineal trauma, sexually transmitted diseases in the premenarchal child, and pregnancy. Anal bleeding, pain on defecation, dysuria, and constipation should also suggest the possibility of abuse. Indirect indicators include unexplained abdominal pain, psychosomatic symptoms or conversion phenomena, secondary bedwetting or faecal soiling, eating disorder, and sleep disturbance. The child

---

Box 6.2 Characteristics of the family of the abused child

- Parents socially isolated
- Parents often drug or alcohol abusers
- Parents were often abused as children
- Parents have unrealistic expectations of parenthood and of the child
- Child often singular, for example through mental or physical handicap
- Family surroundings unsatisfactory, for instance overcrowded
- Abuse begins at times of added parental stress, for example bereavement, redundancy

---

may have a history of running away from home, truancy, poor school performance, or promiscuity.

Where abuse is suspected referral must be made immediately to the local child-abuse team or paediatricians wherever possible; the child may only be willing to tell her story once, and an accurate interview may also need specialist skills such as the use of dolls to help the child re-enact any episodes.

The parent should be interviewed separately before the child is seen, and his or her statement recorded verbatim. On interview the child may seem regressed or inappropriately mature; she should be reassured that she will be believed and not punished for talking. Questions posed should be simple and direct, in order to get an exact picture of what happened and when, including ejaculation.

Examination should begin with inspection of the clothing for blood or staining and a general physical check, as up to three-quarters of sexually abused children show evidence of other abuse (see Box 6.3).

The genital examination follows the guidance above. Genital fondling may not leave physical evidence. Acute changes may include redness, swelling, and abrasions. Scarring or rounding of the hymen and abnormal vulval pigmentation may result long-term. Penetration results in hymenal damage,

---

Box 6.3 Physical indicators of abuse

- Child withdrawn, watchful, avoids eye contact
- Multiple injuries of different ages and types
- Injury of a scale or type inappropriate to the history
- Bruising suggests finger marks or is in a regular distribution
- Specific lesions, including: bites, strap marks, epilation, straight-edge burns, bruising of the pinna, bilateral black eyes, subconjunctival or vitreous haemorrhage, rupture of the frenum labii superioris, extensive facial bruising.

---

pubococcygeal spasm, and external abrasions and laceration. Such injuries lie usually between '3 o'clock' and '9 o'clock' in the supine position. Chronic signs of penetration include hymenal scarring and rounding, widening of the introitus, and pubococcygeal laxity. Anal penetration results in anal tears, initial laxity followed by anal spasm, and pain on defecation which persists after the spasm has relaxed. Chronic abuse results in laxity, anal tags, scarring, and unusual pigmentation.

Specimens for sperm detection and other evidence of abuse or attack should be collected by the child-abuse team in cooperation with the police forensic medical service. Any local injuries should be treated. Emergency contraception may be indicated in the post-menarchal adolescent. Follow-up must be arranged for checking for sexually transmitted infection. The case must be reported to the social services and police, and a place of safety will be needed immediately if the abuser is a member of the family. Psychological follow-up will be needed for both child and family.

Further reading

Baker, A. and Duncan, S. (1986). Child sexual abuse. In *Recent Advances in Paediatrics*, Vol. 8 (ed. R. Meadow), pp. 259–80. Churchill Livingstone, Edinburgh.

Keith Edmonds, D. (1989). *Dewhurst's practical paediatric and adolescent gynaecology*. Butterworth, London.

Muram, D. (1990). Vaginal bleeding in childhood and adolescence. *Obstetrics and Gynaecology Clinics of North America*, **17** (2), 389–408.

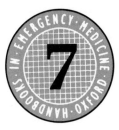

CHAPTER 7

Emergencies relating to contraception

Key points in emergencies relating to contraception

1 Patients must be told of the limitations of postcoital contraception, their informed consent to the method must be recorded formally, and a follow-up family planning appointment must be made for three weeks after their attendance.

2 The patient should be advised to use barrier methods of contraception, or refrain from coitus, for the rest of her cycle as postcoital contraception used early in the cycle may delay ovulation.

Postcoital contraception

• **Oestrogen-based pills   IUCD insertion**

Whether or not postcoital contraception is offered by an individual emergency department is a matter of local policy. The common usage of the name 'morning-after pill' has led to the belief among the public that postcoital hormonal contraception is only effective if taken within a few hours of intercourse, whereas the need to initiate treatment within seventy-two hours of intercourse actually allows considerably more leeway. Some departmental heads therefore believe that postcoital contraception is a primary-care responsibility which it is inappropriate for their department to offer. Other departmental heads feel that they should provide a safety-net for those people who are away from home, are not registered with a general practitioner, or have difficulty accessing their general practitioner with the appropriate degree of urgency.

Whether postcoital contraception is offered through the emergency department or through the primary-care services, it is imperative that the patient is accurately informed of the limitations of the treatment and that follow-up arrangements are made.

Either oestrogen-based pills or intra-uterine contraceptive device insertion may be offered to the patient requesting postcoital contraception.

The most popular hormonal method is the **combined ethinyloestradiol and l-norgestrel pill**. The pill is thought to work by a combination of disruption of the pituitary–ovarian axis and direct action at ovarian and endometrial levels. The luteal phase may be shortened. The endometrium is made hostile to implantation by alteration of the endometrial biochemistry and glandular and stromal development. This is thought to be the main mechanism of action. The pill is therefore a contraceptive agent, in that it prevents implantation, rather than an abortifacient. This distinction may be of great importance in discussion with patients, some of whom would accept contraception but refuse abortion.

Treatment must be initiated within 72 hours of the unprotected intercourse. Two doses are given, to be taken twelve hours apart. The major side-effects associated with the combined pill are nausea (up to 66 per cent), and vomiting (up to 24 per cent).

Reported failure rates range between 0 and 5 per cent. Menses commence within 21 days of the administration of the pill in 98 per cent of women. It is therefore vital that follow-up should be arranged at three weeks after the administration. If menstruation has not occurred, pregnancy-testing is performed at this check. Whilst a large proportion of women experience menstruation earlier than usual, the onset is delayed in some 7 per cent. The patient should be reassured that this may occur and does not necessarily mean contraceptive failure. It must, however, be impressed on all patients that they must keep their three-week appointment.

The emergency physician must discuss with the patient the possibility that the pill may fail. Whilst the majority of patients would opt for a termination in this eventuality, some would not. Whilst oestrogens are known to be terato-genic (an example is diethylstilboestrol), such effects follow multi-dose regimes in early pregnancy, and there is so far no hard evidence of an adverse effect of combined-pill post-coital contraception on the surviving fetus. The teratogenic risk is thought to be smaller than that of continuing the ordinary combined contraceptive pill in early pregnancy. The patient should not be told that she must not accept postcoital contraception unless she intends to proceed to termination in the event of pregnancy. She must, however, be warned that there is such a risk, albeit small; and this warning must be recorded.

Future birth-control methods must be discussed with the patient. Her long-term intentions may be left for discussion at the follow-up appointment. In the short term, she must be warned to use barrier methods, or to refrain from coitus, for the rest of her cycle, as postcoital contraception used early in the cycle may delay ovulation.

Finally, she must be warned that, as it prevents uterine implantation, the postcoital pill will not prevent (indeed some authors think it may encourage) ectopic implantation. Should she develop iliac fossa pain, she must immediately seek medical advice.

The emergency physician must record that the above points have been included in the counselling of the patient, and the patient must be asked to sign a consent form, agreeing that she has been so counselled.

The **intra-uterine contraceptive device (IUCD)** may also be used postcoitally. Again its effect in this context is to prevent implantation. It should be used within 5 days of the date of ovulation. Failures are very rare. Pain is associated with IUCD insertion, and may be of an unacceptable level in the nulliparous. Local anaesthesia may be used. Pre-existing pelvic infection may be exacerbated, and new infection encouraged. IUCD insertion is followed by irregular bleeding *per vaginam*. This may mask early pregnancy; follow-up assessment is therefore essential, despite the very low failure rate of this method. Indications and relative contraindications for postcoital IUCD use are summarized in Box 7.1.

Contraceptive pill overdose

It is not unusual for a parent to consult the emergency department because his or her **child has helped himself or herself to a contraceptive pill**. They may be reassured that there will be no ill effects on a boy, but that a small oestrogen-withdrawal bleed may follow in a girl. This warning must be coupled with reassurance that there are no long-term consequences for the child, that her hormonal balance is not other than temporarily upset, and that the bleed itself will do no harm to the uterus.

Some patients present having taken a deliberate **overdosage of contraceptive pills**, often in combination with other medications and/or alcohol. No major ill effect will result from an overdose of oestrogen, combined, or progesterone-containing pills. Short-term there may be nausea and general malaise. Once the hormone levels drop, menstruation will ensue, and will be heavier than usual.

Box 7.1 **The use of the IUCD for postcoital contraception**

Indications for IUCD use
- Oral contraception contraindicated.
- Patient has presented more than 72 hours post-coitus.
- The patient has had multiple exposures (provided no more than 120 hours have elapsed since the likely time of ovulation).
- The patient wants the most effective method.
- The patient wishes to adopt an IUCD as long-term contraception.
- The patient has vomited the oral postcoital contraceptive.

Relative contraindications
- Nullipara.
- Patient has multiple sexual partners
- Pelvic inflammatory disease.

Further reading

Elstein, M. (1991). Post-coital contraception. In *Handbook of family planning* (2nd edn) (ed. N. Loudon), pp. 269–83. Churchill Livingstone, Edinburgh.

PART 3
The assessment and management of the patient where pregnancy is suspected

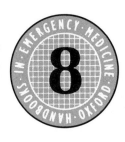

CHAPTER 8

The pregnant patient presenting with bleeding *per vaginam*

Further reading 112

Cross-references:

Key points in bleeding in pregnancy

1 Bleeding in pregnancy may be life-threatening and occult, particularly in ectopic pregnancy, where rupture may cause torrential intra-abdominal bleeding, or in abruption of the placenta, where all or part of the haemorrhage may be concealed.

2 A bleeding pregnant woman near term is able to lose 35 per cent of her circulating volume before showing clinical signs of shock, but the fetus will be compromised as soon as significant haemorrhage starts.

3 The emergency physician must approach the assessment of vaginal bleeding with expedition and care. Fluid resuscitation must be early and vigorous. If the patient is shocked transfusion with group-specific or O-negative blood must be started immediately.

4 The great majority of patients with ectopic pregnancy present a non-acute picture of recurrent lower abdominal pain, irregular vaginal bleeding, and transient syncopal symptoms.

5 Products of conception distending the cervical os may cause hypotension in an aborting patient by a vagal effect. They must be pulled through with ring forceps.

6 Vaginal examination is contra-indicated in patients presenting with ante-partum haemorrhage until ultrasound examination has excluded placenta praevia.

Bleeding during pregnancy may be life-threatening, particularly so in the case of ectopic pregnancy, where rupture may cause torrential intra-abdominal bleeding, or that of abruption of the placenta, where part of the haemorrhage is concealed.

The emergency physician **MUST** approach the assessment of vaginal bleeding with the same expedition and care as expended on any other type of haemorrhage. The first stage is the clinical evaluation of the extent of blood loss (see Chapter 1) and the prompt resuscitation of the patient with intravenous fluids as appropriate. It must be remembered that the plasma volume increases by 50 per cent during pregnancy, and that a bleeding pregnant woman shunts blood away from the utero-placental circulation, thus being able to lose up to 35 per cent of her circulating volume before showing the clinical signs of shock, but compromising the fetus as soon as significant haemorrhage starts. Vigorous fluid infusion and early blood transfusion must be instituted.

High-flow oxygen must be routinely administered to any pregnant woman with other than trivial bleeding.

Supine hypotension, which results from compression of the inferior vena cava by the gravid uterus, must be avoided by nursing the patient on her left side or by elevating the right buttock and displacing the uterus to the left manually.

When abruption of the placenta is suspected, baseline laboratory measurements must include clotting studies and urea and electrolytes, as disseminated intravascular coagulopathy and acute tubular necrosis are associated. Disseminated intravascular coagulopathy is also associated with missed abortion, sepsis, and trophoblastic disease.

The Rh D status of the patient must be known. If antenatal testing has not yet established the mother's blood group, and whether she has immune anti-D if she is Rh D negative, then those tests must be performed in the emergency department. Where the mother is not D-immune, anti-D Ig must be given after birth when the child is Rh D positive, after abortion, ante-partum haemorrhage, and abdominal trauma, and where there is a threatened abortion or suspected ectopic pregnancy. After 20 weeks' gestation, a Kleihauer screening test must be performed to indicate the extent of transplacental haemorrhage (TPH), as high doses of anti-D will be needed if TPH exceeds 4 ml: 250 IU are given before 20 weeks' gestation and 500 IU after twenty weeks, by deep intramuscular injection within 72 hours of the event.

Box 8.1 outlines the approach to the differential diagnosis

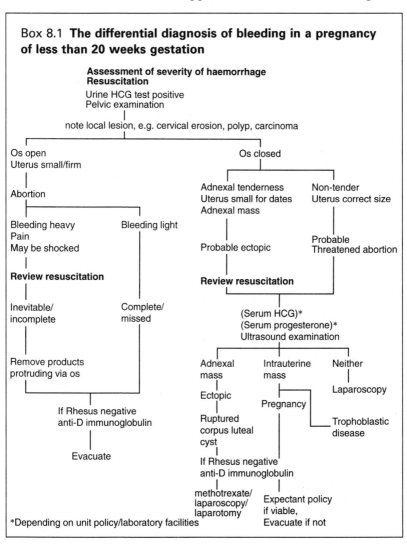

Box 8.1 The differential diagnosis of bleeding in a pregnancy of less than 20 weeks gestation

Assessment of severity of haemorrhage
Resuscitation
Urine HCG test positive
Pelvic examination
note local lesion, e.g. cervical erosion, polyp, carcinoma

Os open
Uterus small/firm

Abortion

Bleeding heavy
Pain
May be shocked

Review resuscitation

Inevitable/
incomplete

Complete/
missed

Bleeding light

Remove products
protruding via os

If Rhesus negative
anti-D immunoglobulin

Evacuate

Os closed

Adnexal tenderness
Uterus small for dates
Adnexal mass

Non-tender
Uterus correct size

Probable ectopic

Probable
Threatened abortion

Review resuscitation

(Serum HCG)*
(Serum progesterone)*
Ultrasound examination

Adnexal
mass

Intrauterine
mass

Neither

Ectopic

Pregnancy

Laparoscopy

Ruptured
corpus luteal
cyst

Trophoblastic
disease

If Rhesus negative
anti-D immunoglobulin

methotrexate/
laparoscopy/
laparotomy

Expectant policy
if viable,
Evacuate if not

*Depending on unit policy/laboratory facilities

of bleeding when the patient is less than twenty weeks pregnant, and Box 8.6 outlines the approach in later pregnancy. The assessment and management of post-partum haemorrhage is detailed in Chapter 13.

The differential diagnosis of bleeding in a pregnancy of less than 20 weeks gestation

The main difficulty in the assessment of vaginal bleeding or pelvic pain presenting in a woman of child-bearing age is the exclusion of ectopic pregnancy, which remains a major cause of maternal death. The symptoms and signs may resemble those of appendicitis, salpingitis, endometriosis, and rupture or torsion of an ovarian cyst. The patient with ectopic implantation may deny amenorrhoea but describe a change of menstrual pattern both in quantity and timing of bleeding over the two or three months preceding presentation; careful questioning is therefore mandatory. A detailed obstetric and gynaecological history should be taken to identify any of the risk factors for ectopia. Box 8.2 lists points to consider in the differential diagnosis between abortion and ectopic.

The finding of a negative HCG urine pregnancy test virtually excludes a viable ectopic pregnancy.

The differential diagnosis to ectopic pregnancy when a positive test is found includes abortion, ruptured corpus luteal cyst of pregnancy, and gestational trophoblastic disease. Ultrasonography is the investigation of choice following HCG testing, the transvaginal approach being particularly valuable in pregnancies of 8 weeks and less. The finding of an intrauterine pregnancy on ultrasound scan excludes ectopic implantation (except in the very rare double pregnancy where one conceptus implants outside the uterine cavity); however, the lack of identification of an adnexal pregnancy on scan does not exclude ectopia. Serum HCG and progesterone levels may have a place in diagnosis, but are outside the remit of most emergency departments.

Appendicitis and ovarian cysts can of course coexist with pregnancy, indeed torsion of ovarian cysts is more common

---

Box 8.2 **Ectopic pregnancy v. threatened abortion: findings on history and examination**

Ectopic	Threatened abortion
Abdominal pain (which may be severe) 96 per cent)	Midline/ crampy pain 10 per cent
Shoulder pain 26 per cent	None
Amenorrhoea 75 per cent	90 per cent
Bleeding *per vaginam* 64 per cent (light)	100 per cent
Shock 17 per cent	None
Dysuria 11 per cent	None
Rectal/defecation pain 9 per cent	None
Passage of decidual cast 7 per cent	None
Abdomen tender 97 per cent 45 per cent generalized 25 per cent bilateral lower quadrants 30 per cent unilateral	Abdomen non-tender
Rebound 60 per cent	None
Adnexal tenderness 94 per cent unilateral 60 per cent	Adnexa non-tender
Adnexal mass 38–50 per cent	None unless luteal cyst
Uterus normal size 80 per cent	Uterus right size for dates

---

during pregnancy. Salpingitis and endometriosis are associated with infertility.

Ectopic pregnancy

Ectopic pregnancy is defined as the implantation of the fertilized ovum elsewhere than in the body of the uterus.

Ectopic implantation occurs in 0.5–1.0 per cent of pregnancies. The incidence is rising. Box 8.3 lists the aetiological conditions.

Box 8.3 **Aetiology of ectopic pregnancy**

- Salpingitis
- Congenital abnormality of conceptus
- Extraneous tubal distortion
- Previous tubal surgery
- IUCD
- Postcoital oestrogen pill or progestin contraceptive pills
- Induction of ovulation using gonadotrophins
- Ovulation dysfunction
- Previous ectopic pregnancy

The main **pathology** underlying ectopic pregnancy is delay in the passage of the ovum to the uterus. At ovulation the egg and its adhering follicular cells are swept into the fallopian tube by the fimbriae and then conducted to the uterus by a combination of muscular contractions and ciliary beating. The adhesions that form following infection or operation may deform the tube: ciliary function may also be damaged. The IUCD is associated with pelvic infection. Uterine, ovarian, or broad ligament tumours and cysts or abdominal surgery may distort the tube. Abnormalities of tract architecture, such as a diverticulum of the tube or a rudimentary horn of the uterus, may lend the ovum a site to implant. Ectopia can follow failed tubal ligation or tubal reanastomosis.

Another mechanism may be disturbance of ovulation and ovum maturation. Ovulation may occur late, leading to withdrawal bleeding before the ovum has a chance to implant. Retrograde menstruation may then force the ovum up the ipsi- or contralateral tube. Corpora lutea contralateral to the pregnancy have been reported. High oestrogen levels from gonadotrophin-induced ovulation may interfere with ovum maturation. Hormonal changes may alter tubal function.

The trophoblast of the ectopic ovum then invades the tubal wall, eroding tubal blood vessels. The resultant decidual reaction in the endosalpinx is patchy and ineffective. Most embryos die within six weeks of implantation owing to this defective placentation. The dead embryo may be reabsorbed, become infected, or mummify. The ovum may implant in the fimbrial, ampullary, infundibular, isthmic, or interstital areas of the fallopian tube (97.7 per cent), in the ovary (0.15 per cent), the broad ligament (0.1 per cent), the abdomen (1.3 per cent), or the cervical or cornual regions of the uterus (0.75 per cent).

The ampulla of the tube is wide and not prone to rupture. The isthmus and interstitial areas are prone to early rupture, being narrow, and the latter to profuse bleeding. Rupture may give rise to a haemoperitoneum; pelvic, broad ligament, or peritubal haematoma; or an abdominal or ligamentary pregnancy. Tubal abortion occurs when the fetus becomes separated from the tubal wall and is extruded into the peritoneal cavity. The abortion may be complete or incomplete. Abdominal or broad ligament pregnancies may result from partial extrusion. If the fetus separates but is not extruded (a missed tubal abortion) it may organize into a tubal mole.

Cornual pregnancies may be extruded into the uterine cavity or may rupture later (at twelve to sixteen weeks), as the horn is distensible. Cervical pregnancies usually abort, and may be accompanied by severe bleeding. Ovarian pregnancies are clinically indistinguishable from those due to rupture of the tube. Abdominal pregnancies usually terminate in the early weeks, but may advance almost to term.

The uterus undergoes the normal response to the hormones of early pregnancy: the organ enlarges, becomes increasingly vascular, softens, and is lined by a mixture of proliferative and secretory endothelium. Once the embryo dies, the decidua is shed, either as fragments or as a cast.

The great majority of cases present with recurrent lower abdominal pain of non-specific nature, amenorrhoea, transient syncopal symptoms, irregular vaginal bleeding (usually slight and dark brown), abdominal tenderness and cervical excitation and vault tenderness on vaginal examination. There may be lower abdominal guarding and rebound tenderness, and a tender adnexal mass may be palpable. The uterus is usually small for the likely gestational age, the majority not feeling clinically enlarged. Softening and bluish discoloration of the cervix may be evident. In the rare interstitial and cornual pregnancies, asymmetrical enlargement of the uterus may be noted. 'Cullen's' sign, of a bruised appearance of the umbilical area, is rare and late. The patient may be pyrexial and may have a leucocytosis.

In a minority of cases the patient presents acutely, with tubal rupture or tubal abortion. The acute picture comprises brief amenorrhoea, severe pain in the iliac fossa or hypogastrium, syncope, shock, and guarding, tenderness and rebound throughout the abdomen. Cervical movement is extremely painful. Where the ovum separates from the tubal wall by chorio-decidual haemorrhage, forming a haematosalpinx, blood may collect around the tube or run down into the rectovaginal pouch (of Douglas). Free intraperitoneal blood may cause shoulder-tip or epigastric pain, and a pelvic haematocele may cause tenesmus, dysuria, and retention, and may be palpable. Occasionally rupture may bring resolution of the pain. **The acutely presenting patient must be vigorously resuscitated** with intravenous fluids and blood, and laparotomy must be promptly performed. It may not be possible to control the bleeding until the damaged tube is exposed.

Where the patient presents a chronic picture, the diagnosis of ectopic pregnancy is difficult, and is only accurate in about half the cases. A urine HCG test will confirm pregnancy, and ultrasound examination using a vaginal probe should reveal the presence of an intrauterine pregnancy, although it may be difficult to interpret the image of a less than six-week fetus. Serial serum β-HCG levels may be used as an indicator of the likelihood of an ectopic pregnancy, a level which increases at less than the usual rate being associated with ectopia. Serum progesterone levels of less than 25 ng/ml have been found to be a sensitive, though non-specific, marker of ectopic pregnancy. Laparoscopy remains an accurate aid to diagnosis, although very early tubal pregnancies may be missed. If the suspected ectopic pregnancy is confirmed, an expectant policy or conservative surgery may be possible in the presence of an early pregnancy. Methotrexate has been advocated by some practitioners. The conservative operator may select laparoscopic salpingostomy, using a laser or cautery; aspiration; manual expression of the ovum; salpingostomy; or segmental resection. Tubal damage may follow a conservative surgical approach, accompanied by an increased risk of recurrent ectopic pregnancy. Other surgeons routinely perform salpingectomy.

Hysterectomy or excision of a uterine horn is indicated for interstitial, cervical, or cornual pregnancies, and salpingo-oophorectomy for ovarian ectopics.

Abdominal pregnancy may be allowed to advance to 32 weeks if viable, when the fetus should be delivered by laparotomy, leaving the placenta *in situ*. Where the fetus has already died, it should be removed at laparotomy.

Sepsis or disseminated intravascular coagulopathy may complicate ectopic pregnancy.

All Rh-negative patients who are not iso-immunized should have Rh immune globulin administered.

Abortion

Abortion is defined as the birth of a non-viable fetus, which is generally held to be one of less than 24 weeks' gestation. Where the abortion is 'threatened' the conceptus is partially detached but viable. When the conceptus is detached the abortion is 'inevitable'. When the conceptus is detached and the products of conception only partially expelled from the uterus the abortion is 'incomplete'. When the conceptus is completely expelled the abortion is 'complete'. When the conceptus has died but the products of conception are retained, the abortion is classed as 'missed'

There is haemorrhage into the decidua basalis, with partial or complete separation of the conceptus, which then stimulates uterine contractions and cervical dilatation. Some 75 per cent of abortions occur before ten weeks' gestation. Abortion is usually complete before six weeks' gestation, and incomplete thereafter until the second trimester. The clinically diagnosed rate is 10–15 per cent. This is an underestimate, as many pregnancies terminate very early.

Box 8.4 lists the aetiological factors.

Box 8.4 **Aetiology of abortion**

- First pregnancy
- Mother aged over 30
- Chromosomal abnormality of the zygotes (50–60 per cent)
- Uterine structural abnormalities
- Cervical incompetence
- Subendometrial fibromyoma
- Maternal disease:—Any severe illness
  —SLE
  —Communicable diseases
  —Uncontrolled diabetes
  —Hypertension
  —Renal disease
  —Thyroid disease
  —Wilson's disease
- Drugs, including isoretinoin, quinine
- High-dose X-ray exposure
- Trauma

The patient has experienced the signs and symptoms of early pregnancy. There is bleeding and may be abdominal pain. Where the abortion is threatened the bleeding is usually light, and pain crampy and mild. Where the conceptus is fully detached bleeding is significant and may be profuse, and the pain may be moderate or severe. If the expulsion of the products of conception is complete, the bleeding will become light. Where the abortion has been missed, the signs and symptoms of pregnancy regress, and there may be episodes of bleeding and pain, a brown discharge, or no loss at all. The conceptus of the missed abortion may organize to form a carneous mole.

On examination the cervix is closed in threatened, open in incomplete, and patulous in complete abortion. The uterus is compatible with the length of gestation in threatened abortion, but is smaller and firmer than expected in incomplete,

complete, or missed abortion. The urine HCG test may be positive in all types of abortion.

The viable fetus of a **threatened abortion** may be confirmed by ultrasound scan. Recent work on serum markers such as Ca-125 has proposed a role for these in predicting the likely outcome of the pregnancy. The traditional advice of bed rest at home and abstinence from coitus has only a minimal effect on the outcome. The value of such advice lies in the emotional support given to the parents in having a practical plan to follow. Around 50 per cent of threatened pregnancies proceed to abort. Light, red blood loss carries a better prognosis than dark-brown. Recurrent or continued loss heralds a poor outcome.

Inevitable and incomplete abortion should be managed by resuscitation with intravenous fluids as necessary and evacuation of the uterus, usually under general anaesthesia and covered by an oxytocin infusion. Such patients may present with hypotension and bradycardia of vasovagal origin and severe pain. If speculum examination reveals products of conception lying in the cervical os, these should be pulled through with ring forceps, thus effecting a rapid improvement in the patient's condition. Removed tissue should be histologically examined. If the patient presents with severe bleeding, ergometrine 500 micrograms is injected intramuscularly and blood transfusion is initiated. Where facilities are limited, evacuation may be effected under local block; or an oxytocin infusion may be started, and the patient transferred as rapidly as possible to the nearest appropriate unit. First-trimester abortions which are apparently complete should be treated as if incomplete.

Missed abortions will eventually be expelled naturally; but evacuation will remove the risk of coagulopathy, and may be better for the parents psychologically. The uterus in such cases is friable and relatively non-contractile. Evacuation under ten weeks' gestation is performed by dilatation and curettage; after ten weeks it may be initiated by prostaglandin E2 intravaginally. Coagulation defects should be sought and blood cross-matched preoperatively. Curettage should be covered by an oxytocin infusion. It may be necessary to proceed to emergency hysterectomy.

Rh negative patients should be given Rh immune globulin if non-immune.

Sepsis may follow spontaneous or surgically induced abortion. The incidence is reported as 5–25 per cent. Pregnancy with an IUCD *in situ* carries a greater risk. The patient may present with vaginal bleeding, pyrexia, tachycardia, and uterine tenderness, or with hypotension and peripheral shutdown. There may be an offensive discharge, peritonitis, or signs of operative trauma. The obstetrician should be immediately involved. *Staphylococcus aureus*, coliforms, *Bacteroides* and *Clostridium welchii* are the usual pathogens. Septic abortion should be treated with broad-spectrum antibiotics given intravenously, after taking blood samples and high vaginal swabs for bacterial culture. Augmentin is a reasonable initial therapy. A baseline full blood count and blood grouping should be requested, as both haemolysis and haemorrhage may occur. A clotting screen should be ordered. A chest X-ray may reveal subdiaphragmatic air from uterine perforation. Once there is good antibiotic cover, the uterus should ideally be evacuated by curettage, covered with an oxytocin infusion if the gestation has passed twelve weeks. However, evacuation may be needed to control bleeding.

Finally, the psychological impact of miscarriage must not be disregarded or underestimated. The parents may suffer a severe bereavement reaction. Self-blame is almost universal, and there may be great fear about the prognosis for any future pregnancies. Reassurance should be offered that the next pregnancy has an 85 per cent chance of proceeding successfully, and (in nearly all cases) that the parents were not in any way responsible for the loss. Some parents derive great comfort from having the miscarried fetus afforded the same rights as a stillbirth, and the emergency team should keep to hand the names of religious practitioners who will offer such a service. Follow-up counselling arrangements are wise, even if these consist only of an interview with the obstetrician to re-rehearse the causes of abortion and the future outlook. Occasionally, immediate psychiatric help may be needed.

Gestational trophoblastic disease

Trophoblastic disease occurs in about 0.05 per cent of gestations in this country, although it is far more common in the developing world. It is more common in women aged less than twenty or more than forty. It is thought to result from either the merger of a haploid sperm with an anucleate oocyte or the fertilization of one oocyte by two sperm (or a diploid sperm). The pathological picture is a spectrum of conditions, from the mass of grape-like vesicles which fill the uterus in hydatidiform mole, through more invasive changes, to the masses of syncytio- and cytotrophoblast which characterize choriocarcinoma. Choriocarcinoma usually follows hydatidiform mole, but may follow abortion, ectopic pregnancy, or normal delivery.

Bleeding *per vaginam* usually commences around the 12th to 16th week of gestation. Excessive vomiting may occur, abdominal pain may be marked, and proteinuria and hypertension are common. The uterus is large for dates in 50 per cent of cases and small in 25 per cent. HCG levels are high, and ultrasound examination has a characteristic 'snowstorm' appearance. The ovaries may be enlarged, and the thyroid gland mildly overactive as a result of the large amounts of HCG which these tumours produce. The hydatidiform mole is often aborted at around 20 weeks, when vesicles may be mixed with the vaginal blood. The abortion is encouraged with syntocinon. Where abortion has not begun the mole is evacuated with suction curettage. All patients should be regularly followed up with clinical examination and urinary HCG estimations for two years.

Choriocarcinoma may present with vaginal bleeding or with the manifestations of metastatic spread. On examination the purplish nodules of vaginal metastases, which are common, may be seen. The tumour invades both blood and lymphatic systems, giving rise to widespread deposits in other organs, including the lung, brain, and kidneys. Chemotherapy has transformed the prognosis for choriocarcinoma, which is now eminently curable. Disseminated intravascular coagulopathy may accompany trophoblastic disease.

The differential diagnosis of bleeding in a pregnancy of more than 20 weeks gestation (ante-partum haemorrhage)

Ante-partum haemorrhage affects 2.5 per cent of pregnancies. As always, the physician's first responsibility is the assessment of the patient's haemodynamic state and rapid resuscitation, with the early use of blood transfusion. **Vaginal examination is contraindicated in the patient who presents with ante-partum haemorrhage.** Baseline measures of full blood count, grouping, and clotting profile should be made. The aetiology is outlined in Box 8.5.

Box 8.5 **Aetiology of ante-partum haemorrhage**

- Unclassified 45 per cent
- Abruptio placentae 30 per cent
- Placenta praevia 20 per cent
- Miscellaneous 5 per cent
  including:
  Cervical polyp
  Cervical cancer
  Vaginal varices
  Vaginitis
  Uterine rupture

The approach to the differential diagnosis of antepartum haemorrhage is summarized in Box 8.6.

Abruptio placentae

Abruptio placentae is defined as the separation of a normally situated placenta after the 20th week of gestation. It affects 0.67 per cent of pregnancies. The aetiology is outlined in Box 8.7.

Box 8.6 **The differential diagnosis of bleeding in a pregnancy of more than 20 weeks gestation**

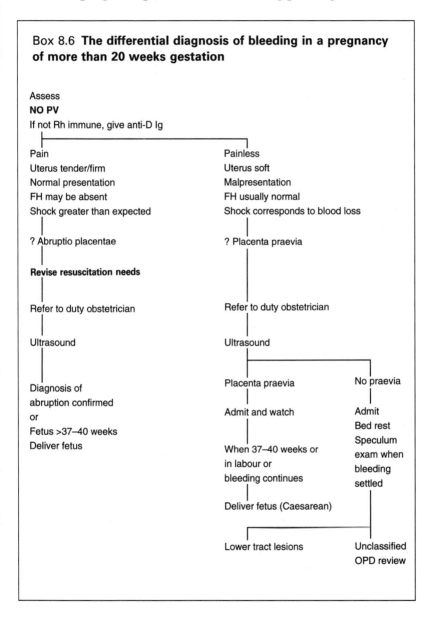

Assess
NO PV
If not Rh immune, give anti-D Ig

Pain	Painless
Uterus tender/firm	Uterus soft
Normal presentation	Malpresentation
FH may be absent	FH usually normal
Shock greater than expected	Shock corresponds to blood loss

? Abruptio placentae   ? Placenta praevia

Revise resuscitation needs

Refer to duty obstetrician   Refer to duty obstetrician

Ultrasound   Ultrasound

Diagnosis of   Placenta praevia   No praevia
abruption confirmed
or   Admit and watch   Admit
Fetus >37–40 weeks   Bed rest
Deliver fetus   Speculum
                                When 37–40 weeks or   exam when
                                in labour or   bleeding
                                bleeding continues   settled

                                Deliver fetus (Caesarean)

                                Lower tract lesions   Unclassified
                                                          OPD review

Box 8.7 **Aetiology of abruptio placentae**

Risk factors include:
- Hypertension (including eclampsia)
- Smoking
- Vitamin deficiency
- Trauma
- Sudden decompression of an over-distended uterus (for example after delivery of a first twin or rupture of the membranes in polyhydramnios)
- Circumvallate placenta
- Previous abruption (11 per cent recurrence rate)

The placental separation is caused by haemorrhage int the decidua basalis. The blood usually tracks down betweei the uterus and membranes to appear externally. This i: termed 'revealed haemorrhage'. Where blood is trapped between the placenta and uterus (10 per cent of cases) extravasation of blood into the myometrium may cause uterine tenderness, pain, and contractions. This is termed 'concealed haemorrhage'. Rarely, blood may dissect through the myometrium, giving intraperitoneal bleeding. Cases where there is both external and retroplacental bleeding are called 'mixed'. Around 50 per cent of cases present before the 36th week of gestation. Most cases present with vaginal bleeding (90 per cent), pain (50 per cent), an irritable uterus, and a localized area of tenderness. If the abruption is posterior the uterine tenderness may be replaced by low back pain. Some cases of the revealed type may mimic placenta praevia in presenting with painless bleeding and a non-tender uterus. In severe concealed haemorrhage the patient presents with severe pain, profound shock, and an acute abdomen. On examination the uterus is hard and tender throughout. No fetal heart sounds are heard.

There is a very real risk of undertransfusing patients with abruptio placentae. Intravenous fluids must be administered immediately, followed by blood transfusion as indicated. When assessing transfusion needs, the association of abruption with hypertension must be remembered; a 'normal' blood pressure in a patient who was hypertensive indicates hypovolaemia. If the patient is shocked 1 to 2 l of blood have already been lost, and transfusion must be performed immediately, either with group-specific or O-negative blood. A catheter must be inserted, and the urine output must be carefully monitored. **Central venous pressure monitoring is indicated wherever a significant degree of bleeding is suspected.** Blood samples must be taken for FBC, clotting studies, and cross-matching (4 units initially) as necessary. The serum marker Ca-125 has been found to be a highly specific and fairly sensitive indicator of abruption.

The maternal vital signs and fundal height must be carefully monitored. The fetus should be continuously monitored. If the bleeding is slight and there is no uterine tenderness, expectant treatment may be pursued.

In all other cases the fetus should be delivered either by amniotomy induction or by Caesarean section. Caesarean section is preferred in more severe cases, where there is fetal distress, or where induction is contraindicated or fails, or labour is progressing inadequately after six hours.

Some 10 per cent of cases of abruption are associated with disseminated intravascular coagulopathy, either in particularly severe cases or where bleeding was concealed. A careful watch must be maintained for bleeding from needle-puncture sites. Where a significant amount of blood has infiltrated the myometrium (the 'Couvelaire' uterus), and DIC occurs, there may be significant post-partum haemorrhage. Renal failure due to cortical and tubular necrosis may follow the hypovolaemia attendant on abruption (see p. 128).

Placenta praevia

Placenta praevia is defined as the siting of the placenta wholly or partly in the lower uterine segment, which is that portion of the uterus below the reflection of the uterovesical peritoneal reflection. It affects 0.5 per cent of births, and is recurrent in 5 per cent of these. The aetiology is outlined in Box 8.8.

Box 8.8 **Aetiology of placenta praevia**

Risk factors include:
- High parity
- Mothers aged over 35
- Placental and cord abnormalities, for example
  —bipartite placenta
  —velamentous insertion of the cord
- Uterine tumours
- Previous uterine incisions
- Multiple pregnancy
- Close-spaced pregnancies
- Previous placenta praevia (increased incidence: ×12)

The lower uterine segment forms towards the end of the second trimester. Accurate judgement of the extent of encroachment of the placenta before this time is therefore not always possible. Four types of praevia are recognized (see Fig. 8.1). Types 1 and 2 make up half the presentations, types 3 and 4 the other 50 per cent. As the lower segment stretches, the placenta may peel off the uterine wall. The great majority of patients therefore present clinically with painless bleeding in the last trimester. Most initially experience a small self-limiting haemorrhage. Bleeding then recurs intermit-

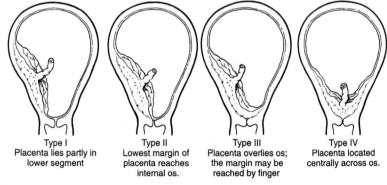

| Type I | Type II | Type III | Type IV |
| Placenta lies partly in lower segment | Lowest margin of placenta reaches internal os. | Placenta overlies os; the margin may be reached by finger | Placenta located centrally across os. |

Fig. 8.1 • Degrees of placenta praevia.

tently, and 90 per cent of patients suffer a significant haemorrhage at some stage, of which up to a quarter result in shock; but 15 per cent of patients do not bleed until labour starts. The uterus is soft and non-tender, and the fetus is usually not distressed. However, the fetus is 'high-riding', and malpresentations are common. The use of routine ultrasound examination during pregnancy leads to many possible cases being identified before they present clinically: 90 per cent of these apparent praevias will resolve as the lower segment develops. In most cases the patient should be admitted and placed on bed rest. The placenta is localized by ultrasound examination, and fetal monitoring is undertaken. The maternal blood loss is treated as appropriate. Where praevia is confirmed, Caesarean section is performed after 37 weeks.

Where labour has commenced, or bleeding is heavy and persistent, or continues intermittently and is accompanied by concern about the well-being of the fetus, Caesarean section should be performed imminently.

The risk of post-partum haemorrhage is increased by placenta praevia, as the lower uterine segment is relatively atonic, and placental adherence is greater than in the upper segment, the decidual response of the lower segment being relatively poor (see 'post-partum haemorrhage', Chapter 13).

Unclassified cases of bleeding

Some cases remain **unclassified**. Some of these cases may be due to minor degrees of abruptio or placenta praevia. Others are thought to be due to the rupture of small blood vessels in the isthmus and cervix. The patient may be mobilized and discharged once the bleeding settles. Perinatal mortality is higher amongst the children of these patients. Close outpatient supervision is required, and induction should be considered after 37 weeks.

Cervical erosions and polyps, or carcinoma, vaginitis, and vulvo-vaginal varices may all cause vaginal bleeding in pregnancy.

Further reading

Ashworth, F. (1992). Septic abortion. In *Spontaneous abortion, diagnosis and treatment* (ed. I. Stabile, J. G. Grudzinskas, and T. Chard), pp. 119–32. Springer-Verlag, Berlin.

Fleming, A. D. (1991). Abruptio placentae. *Critical Care Clinics*, **7** (4), 865–75.

Mabie, W. C. (1992). Placenta praevia. *Clinics in Perinatology*, **19** (2), 425–35.

National Blood Transfusion Service Immunoglobulin Working Party (1991). Recommendations for the use of anti-D immunoglobulin. *Prescriber's Journal*, **31** (4), 137–45.

Nielson, E. C., Varner, M. W., and Scott, J. R. (1991). The outcome of pregnancy complicated by bleeding during the second trimester. *Surgery, Gynaecology and Obstetrics*, **173** (5), 371–4.

Ory, S. J. (1992). New options for diagnosis and treatment of ectopic pregnancy. *Journal of the American Medical Association*, **267** (4), 534–7.

Stabile, I., Campbell, S., and Grudzinskas, J. G. (1989). Ultrasound and circulating placental protein measurements in complications of early pregnancy. *British Journal of Obstetrics and Gynaecology*, **96** (10), 1182–91.

Stabile, I., Grudzinskas, J. G., and Chard, T. (ed.) (1992). *Spontaneous abortion: Diagnosis and treatment*. Springer-Verlag, Berlin.

Stovall, T. G., Keelerman, A. L., Ling, F. W., and Buster, J. E. (1990). Emergency Department diagnosis of ectopic pregnancy. *Annals of Emergency Medicine*, **19** (10), 1098–103.

Weckstein, L. N. (1987). Clinical diagnosis of ectopic pregnancy. *Clinical Obstetrics and Gynecology*, **30** (1), 236–44.

Witt, B. R., Wolf, G. C., Wainwright, C. J., Johnston, P. D. and Thorneycroft, I. H. (1990). Relaxin, Ca-125, progesterone, estradiol, Schwangerschaft protein, and HCG as predictors of outcome in threatened and non-threatened pregnancies. *Fertility and Sterility*, **53** (6), 1029–36.

Witt, B. R., Miles, R., Wolf, G. C., Koulianos, G. T., and Thorneycroft, I. H. (1991). Ca-125 levels in abruptio placenta. *American Journal of Obstetrics and Gynecology*, **164** (5, part 1), 1225–8.

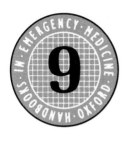

CHAPTER 9

The pregnant patient presenting with abdominal pain

Key points in abdominal pain in pregnancy

1 Surgery is usually well-tolerated in pregnancy, and may be life-saving. Misdiagnosis and delay in treatment of non-obstetric abdominal pathology carry significant maternal and fetal morbidity and mortality.

2 Diagnostic imaging should, where possible, be non-irradiative or use the lowest possible radiation dose, however X-ray studies should not be withheld where they are needed for diagnosis.

3 Complications of ovarian masses are more common in the pregnant than the non-pregnant patient. Torsion is always an indication for immediate operation, even where the pregnancy is advanced.

4 In early pregnancy, the presentation of acute appendicitis resembles that in the non-pregnant patient, but the appendix is displaced upwards by the growing uterus until, by term, the pain of appendicitis is localized to the right flank.

5 Intestinal obstruction may be missed as its symptoms of nausea, vomiting, and constipation are common concomitants of pregnancy itself.

6 Acute pyelonephritis is common in pregnancy and causes very significant fetal and maternal morbidity. The presenting picture is variable and often non-specific. A high level of suspicion must be maintained.

The previous chapter details the diagnosis and early management of ectopic pregnancy, abortion, and abruption of the placenta, conditions characteristically accompanied by pain as well as bleeding.

Up to 2 per cent of pregnancies may be complicated by non-obstetric abdominal pathology requiring operative intervention. Surgery is usually well tolerated in pregnancy, and may be life-saving. Misdiagnosis and delay in treatment carry significant maternal and fetal morbidity and mortality. Misdiagnosis may result from a lack of appreciation of the bulk effect of the pregnant uterus on the positions of intra-abdominal structures and of the physiological changes which accompany gestation (see Chapter 16). Nausea, vomiting, constipation or diarrhoea, and urinary symptoms are common enough in normal pregnancy; but they should arouse suspicion when they appear suddenly and whenever they are accompanied by pain.

There may also be reluctance to use imaging to confirm a suspected diagnosis. Fetal exposure of less than 5 rads is unlikely to lead to any congenital abnormalities, and lead shields can be used to protect the uterus. Consideration can be given to using imaging techniques, such as ultrasound, which do not involve irradiation; to selecting the lowest irradiation technique (for instance, avoid fluoroscopy); and to limiting the number of exposures taken during a study; but where X-ray studies are needed they must be performed promptly, pregnancy or no. The need for the investigations must be explained to the patient, and she must be reassured that their performance is in her baby's best interest. The patient presenting with hypovolaemic shock or peritonitis must be energetically resuscitated with intravenous fluids. The woman in the third trimester of pregnancy has the reserve of her 50 per cent increase in plasma volume to cushion haemorrhage, and will not show the classic signs and symptoms of shock until she has lost a third of her circulating volume. The fetus has no such cushion, and will suffer from a decreased blood supply as soon as there is significant maternal bleeding. This disparity between appearance and need of the mother and fetus is the linchpin of effective fluid replacement, which must be based on an estimate of losses and the response of the mother's central venous pressure to infusion. The fetus must be monitored. Generalized peritonitis must be managed with fluids, antibiotics, and expeditious laparotomy.

The differential diagnosis of pelvic pain in pregnancy

Box 9.1 details the approach to the differential diagnosis of pelvic pain.

The presentations of ectopic pregnancy, abortion and abruption of the placenta are discussed in Chapter 8.

Complications of ovarian masses are a common cause of severe abdominal pain in pregnancy. Corpus luteal cysts, dermoid cysts, and serous cystadenomas are the league leaders. Up to 5 per cent of ovarian tumours of the pregnant patient are malignant. Torsion is more common in the pregnant patient than in the non-pregnant; estimates of the rate of torsion of ovarian masses during pregnancy vary from 10 per cent to 60 per cent. The peak incidences are during the first trimester and post-partum. Up to 5 per cent of ovarian cysts rupture during pregnancy, often during labour.

Treatment (of cysts) should not be denied the pregnant patient, although deferment beyond the 16th week of pregnancy is desirable if possible. **Torsion is always an indication for immediate operation, even where the pregnancy is advanced.**

Red degeneration of a uterine fibromyoma occurs when there is vascular resupply of a fibroid that has undergone fatty degeneration. It usually occurs during pregnancy, and presents with pain and enlargement and tenderness of the uterine mass. It may be treated conservatively with pain-relief and rest.

Acute polyhydramnios is a rare condition associated with uniovular twins, where excess amniotic fluid accumulates quickly. The patient presents with abdominal pain and vomiting. The abdomen is large for the length of gestation,

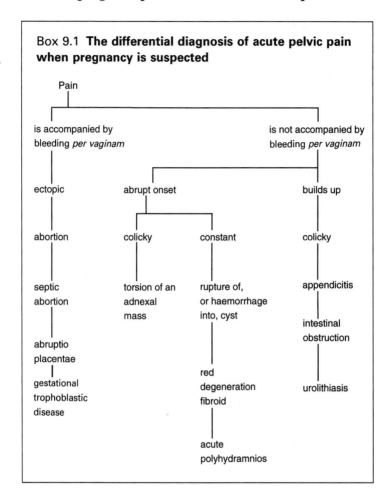

Box 9.1 **The differential diagnosis of acute pelvic pain when pregnancy is suspected**

the wall is stretched and may be oedematous, and the fetal heart sounds muffled. The uterus is very tense; a fluid thrill can be elicited. The fetus is unusually mobile. The patient should be referred to the obstetrician: labour is induced if the fetus is near term; amniocentesis may relieve the pain where gestation is not so advanced.

The differential diagnosis of upper abdominal pain in pregnancy

The differential diagnosis of upper abdominal pain presenting in pregnancy is summarized in Box 9.2.

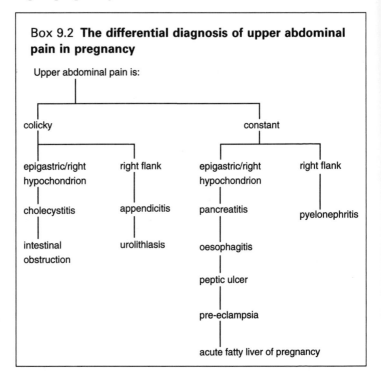

Box 9.2 **The differential diagnosis of upper abdominal pain in pregnancy**

Upper abdominal pain is:

colicky

    epigastric/right hypochondrion → cholecystitis → intestinal obstruction

    right flank → appendicitis → urolithiasis

constant

    epigastric/right hypochondrion → pancreatitis → oesophagitis → peptic ulcer → pre-eclampsia → acute fatty liver of pregnancy

    right flank → pyelonephritis

Pre-eclampsia is discussed in Chapter 12 and acute fatty liver of pregnancy is discussed in Chapter 10.

Non-obstetric causes of abdominal pain in pregnancy

Cholelithiasis and cholecystitis are more commonly found in the pregnant than the non-pregnant woman, owing to the relative bile stasis resulting from progesterone-led smooth-muscle relaxation and to alterations in the cholesterol–bile salt ratio. Multiparous women and those in the late stages of pregnancy are particularly at risk. The symptoms of chole-cystitis are the same as in the non-pregnant patient. The uterus, however, displaces the gall-bladder upwards, so that it comes to lie under the right costal margin. Ultrasonography should confirm the diagnosis. The patient should be referred for admission, and, initially, conservative care. Unless the severity of the patient's condition demands early surgery, many practitioners prefer to operate post-parturition.

Intestinal obstruction during pregnancy is usually due to the presence of postoperative adhesions, although volvulus (especially that of the sigmoid colon), strangulated hernia, intussusception, and mesenteric thrombosis may occur. Most cases present in late pregnancy, particularly when the head engages, or during the early post-partum period. Nausea, vomiting, and constipation are not rare in pregnancy, and the diagnosis may not be suspected. The presentation of obstruction is similar to that in the non-pregnant patient. Examination reveals hyperactive 'tinkling' bowel sounds, and fluid levels can be seen on the plain abdominal film. A 'drip-and-suck' regime is instituted, and the patient is admitted. Surgery is offered if a conservative regime does not resolve the condition.

The presentation of **appendicitis** in early pregnancy parallels that in the non-pregnant patient. The characteristic presentation is very like that of ectopic pregnancy, see Chapter 8. As pregnancy advances, whilst the initial pain from the distended, inflamed appendix is felt in the peri-umbilical area, the localized tenderness resulting from inflammation of the peritoneum overlying the appendix is displaced cranially, coming to lie in the right flank by term. Rectal and vaginal examination usually reveal right-sided tenderness. Secondary inflammation of the urinary tract may cause pyuria and microscopic haematuria, which may be misleading. The incidence of perforation is higher in the pregnant than in the non-pregnant woman. Surgical intervention is urgently indicated to minimize both maternal and fetal danger.

Urolithiasis is rare in pregnancy. The symptomatology is characteristic: the patient is afebrile, and urinalysis reveals haematuria rather than pyuria. Intravenous pyelography should be avoided if possible; ultrasonography is the investigation of choice. Treatment is as conservative as possible, the patient being admitted for fluids, analgesia, and antibiotic cover as indicated.

Pancreatitis in pregnancy is probably largely related to the incidence of gallstones. It may also complicate preeclampsia and acute fatty liver. The patient presents with constant epigastric pain radiating to the back, often accompanied by nausea, vomiting, and pyrexia. On examination the abdomen is distended and bowel sounds are decreased (in late pregnancy bowel sounds should be assessed over the upper abdomen). Hypotension and peritonism may be found. Serum amylase is usually raised; there may be hypocalcaemia; and electrolyte studies will reflect hypovolaemia, and may herald the onset of renal failure. Hyperglycaemia occurs. A drip-and-suck regime is instituted, and the patient should be admitted for rehydration, treatment of hyperglycaemia and hypocalcaemia, and pain-relief. Prophylactic antibiotics may be added to the regime. Maternal and fetal mortality are high in this condition.

Peptic ulceration usually improves during pregnancy, whilst **oesophageal reflux** pain is almost standard during the last trimester. Patients who give a history of previous ulcers, or where there is a strong clinical suspicion, may be offered endoscopy and/or treated with H2 blockers and antacids as indicated. Perforation may occur, particularly during the third trimester. Immediate surgery is indicated.

Acute pyelonephritis is a common complication of pregnancy, due to the ureteral dilatation and urinary stasis which accompany the condition. Inadequately treated it may lead to abortion or intrauterine death, fetal growth retardation, premature labour, or chronic pyelonephritis, leading to hypertension and renal failure. The patient with a history of childhood urine infections or any structural abnormality of the renal tract is at increased risk, and a finding of bacteruria in an asymptomatic patient is an indication for prophylactic treatment. It presents, usually after the sixteenth week of gestation, with lumbar or loin pain, fever, frequency of urination, and dysuria. Vomiting and rigors may occur. The former may in some cases be the predominant and presenting symptom. The right kidney is involved in 85 per cent of cases, 35 per cent being unilateral. The left kidney is unilaterally involved in only 15 per cent. Examination, which is best performed in the lateral position with the affected side uppermost, reveals significant pyrexia, tachycardia, and tenderness over the kidney, but is unlikely to reveal peritonism. Urine examination shows white, red, and epithelial cells, proteinuria, and bacteria, and culture grows *E. coli* in 80 per cent of cases. Intravenous ampicillin 500 mg IV four times a day should be started as soon as the MSU sample has been taken if pyuria is present. The patient should be admitted for rest, pain-relief, and the continuation of antibiotic therapy based on the cultured organism.

The onset of the condition may be more gradual, with a lesser fever but other characteristic symptoms, or the patient may present with an isolated complaint of vomiting, pain, or rigors. The emergency physician must maintain a high level of suspicion and examine the urine in any case of vomiting after the first trimester or of unexplained pyrexia.

Further reading

Richards, C. and Daya, S. (1989). Diagnosis of acute appendicitis in pregnancy. *Canadian Journal of Surgery*, **32** (5), 358–60.

Rubin, S. C. (1989). Acute abdominal pain in pregnancy. In *Obstetric emergencies* (ed. G. Benrubi), pp. 25–44. Churchill Livingstone, Edinburgh.

Tamir, I. L., Bongard, F. S., and Klein, S. R. (1990). Acute appendicitis in the pregnant patient. *American Journal of Surgery*, **160** (6), 571–6.

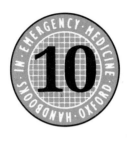

CHAPTER 10

The pregnant patient with intercurrent disease

Dermatological conditions 141

Communicable disease 141

Dependency 146

Psychiatric disease 146

Further reading 147

Key points in the pregnant patient with intercurrent disease

1 All pregnant women with a blood pressure above 140/90 mmHg or proteinuria should be referred for consideration of admission to hospital.

2 Most cases of renal failure due to obstetric causes will respond rapidly and well to the reversal of hypovolaemia.

3 Status asthmaticus should be treated in accordance with standard treatment protocols.

4 If heart failure supervenes in a pregnant patient, the use of morphine, diuretics, and vasodilators follows standard practice.

5 45 per cent of pregnant epileptic patients suffer an increased frequency of fitting. The onset of fitting after 20 weeks gestation is indicative of eclampsia. A raised blood pressure accompanying a fit in the second half of pregnancy should be treated as eclampsia.

6 Patients with infective hepatitis may be asymptomatic or have non-specific symptoms. 50 per cent of babies born vaginally, but only 5 per cent of those delivered by Caesarean section, to those infected will be B Ag-positive and may develop hepatic carcinoma or chronic active hepatitis.

7 Acute fatty liver of pregnancy presents with upper abdominal pain and vomiting. It is a dire condition.

8 Diabetic ketoacidosis develops at lower blood glucose levels than those usually found in the condition. Fetal death results in more than half the cases.

9 Thyroid storm may accompany labour, pre-eclampsia, or trauma. If the clinical picture is suggestive, treatment should be commenced without awaiting laboratory investigations.

10 No woman should commence labour with a haemoglobin level below 10 g/dl. If a significantly anaemic woman presents in labour, blood transfusion with packed cells under diuretic cover is required.

11 Septic shock is a dire emergency for mother and child. If the origin of the infection cannot quickly be identified, treatment should commence on the assumption that the parent infection is pelvic.

12 Staff should take routine precautions against infection with HIV when delivering children. Specific procedures should be followed for the delivery of the babies of mothers in high-risk groups.

13 Any pregnant woman with a non-specific pyrexia of over 38 degrees which has persisted for 48 hours, must be treated as infected with listeria.

14 If a baby born to a chronic opiate addict starts sneezing, withdrawal symptoms are starting and the infant should be given oral chlorpromazine immediately.

15 Haloperidol 10–30 mg IM or chlorpromazine 25–50 mg IM are reasonable first choices for control of the acutely psychotic pregnant patient.

Hypertension

Blood pressure should be measured with the mother semi-prone in the first two trimesters, and in the lateral position, with the sphygnomanometer cuff at the level of the heart, in the third trimester. A blood pressure above 140/90 in the first twenty weeks of pregnancy is likely to reflect pre-existing disease rather than pregnancy-related hypertension. About a third of women with chronic hypertension have a further rise of blood pressure during pregnancy. The woman with a history of chronic hypertension is five times more likely to develop pre-eclampsia when pregnant than a woman without such a history. A rise of 30 mmHg in the systolic level, or 15 mmHg in the diastolic level, compared to previous readings, indicates that pre-eclampsia may be supervening. The management of pre-eclampsia is outlined in Chapter 12.

In all cases the baby should be delivered as soon as the fetus is mature (37 weeks); but delivery will be imperative earlier in cases where the disease is more severe, there being a low threshold for Caesarean section. All pregnant women with hypertension above 140/90 mmHg or proteinuria should be admitted to hospital, the hypertension being initially treated by rest.

Whilst most patients have essential hypertension, renal, vascular, and endocrine causes must be considered, and assessment of renal size and radio-femoral delay, examination of the urine, and measurement of urea and creatinine levels must be undertaken. Renal disease carries a serious prognosis, and phaeochromocytoma, although rare, leads to significant mortality. A phaeochromocytoma may present with the classic paroxysmal attack of hypertension, tachycardia, pallor, headache, sweating, and vomiting, or with sustained hypertension. Labour, delivery, anaesthesia, and surgery are liable to precipitate attacks, which may cause cardiac failure and death. Urine catecholamines and vanillyl mandelic acid are raised. Caesarean section is the preferred method of delivery. Intravenous phentolamine will control the acute attack.

Renal disease

Abruptio placentae, eclampsia, septic abortion, and post-partum haemorrhage may all give rise to acute renal failure, i.e. to a fall in glomerular filtration rate over hours/days, often associated with oliguria. Occasionally, acute renal failure may follow an apparently normal pregnancy and delivery.

Usually, renal histology shows acute tubular necrosis, a recoverable condition; but sometimes there is pathology of small arterioles in combination with a haemolytic state ('haemolytic–uraemic syndrome'). The latter condition, if severe, may lead to cortical necrosis, a condition which is not completely recoverable. The management of acute renal failure is summarized in Box 10.1. Most obstetric cases will respond rapidly and well to the reversal of hypovolaemia.

The commonest causes of chronic renal failure in women of child-bearing age are the various forms of glomerulonephritis, reflux nephropathy, and diabetic nephropathy. Patients should be carefully followed through pregnancy, and admitted if their blood pressure becomes unacceptably high or their renal function deteriorates.

There may be fetal growth retardation and increased risk of perinatal death, especially in patients who are hypertensive. It is usual to ensure delivery by the 38th week of gestation at the latest.

Urinary tract infections, which are more common in patients with renal failure than in the general pregnant population, should be sought and treated. Symptomatic urinary tract infections should be treated with the appropriate antibacterial agent. Common infecting organisms are E. coli, Klebsiella, and Proteus. Amoxycillin (or ampicillin) 500 mg three times a day, trimethoprim 200 mg twice a day, or cephelexin 500 mg four times a day may be used. A five-day course should be given. The patient should be advised to take copious fluids, and follow-up must be arranged to revise treatment in the light of microbial culture sensitivities. If there are relapses the underlying cause should be sought.

Acute pyelonephritis is an important condition in preg-

Box 10.1 **Management of acute renal failure**

- Check clotting profile, urea and electrolytes, plasma albumen, blood gases, urinalysis, BP.
- Assess hypovolaemia clinically, monitor CVP.
- Correct hypovolaemia using colloid.
- Correct acidosis using crystalloids.
- Infuse dopamine at 1–3 micrograms/kg/min.
- Infuse dobutamine if the systolic BP is less than 100 mmHg.
- Give as a bolus 120 mg frusemide. If no diuresis results, give a further 250–500 mg.
- Treat K+ greater than 6.5 mmol with 20 ml of 10 per cent calcium gluconate, 50–100 ml of 8.4 per cent sodium bicarbonate, dextrose/insulin infusion of 50 ml of 50 per cent dextrose with 16 units of soluble 'human' insulin over 30 minutes.
- If diuresis does not occur give fluids hourly on the basis of replacing measured losses plus estimated insensible losses.
- Commence antibiotics if the cause is thought to be septic.
- Renal ultrasound should be performed at the earliest opportunity.
- The patient should be admitted to an obstetric unit in a hospital with dialysis facilities and expertise.

---

nancy. It presents with fever, malaise, headache, loin pain and, sometimes, rigors. There may be NO lower urinary tract symptoms. Mid-stream urine examination should be diagnostic. The patient should be admitted for parenteral antibiotics and fluids. Further details of the condition may be found in Chapter 9.

Preterm labour is associated with urinary tract infection. Where there is pyuria without bacteruria, chlamydial infection may be present. Patients with these symptoms who have neither pyuria nor bacteruria must be followed up and re-evaluated within two weeks.

Renal failure, proteinuria, and hypertension are important manifestations of systemic lupus erythematosus. In some patients with 'lupus anticoagulant' *in vitro* there is a thrombotic tendency *in vivo*. Placental clotting may result in fetal death, and phlebothrombosis may lead to pulmonary embolism.

Polycystic disease of the kidneys affects 1:1000 of the population. The large kidneys do not usually interfere with the pregnancy, but many patients are hypertensive, and some may have renal impairment. Patients with polycystic disease have a higher incidence of urinary tract infection. The disease is autosomal dominant, and may be detected on chromosome studies in early pregnancy. Such patients should be encouraged to seek genetic counselling if they have not already done so.

Respiratory disease

Asthma may appear to worsen (25 per cent of cases) or improve (25 per cent of cases) during pregnancy. Provided fetal oxygenation is ensured, there is no increased perinatal morbidity or mortality.

Status asthmaticus should be treated in accordance with usual asthmatic protocols. Chest X-ray with abdominal shielding will expose the fetus to minimal radiation, and should be performed to exclude infection or a pneumothorax. Oxygen and fluids are administered. Nebulized beta sympathetomimetics and atropine may be used. There is no contraindication to intravenous or oral glucocorticoids (for example hydrocortisone 1 g per 24 hrs); the increased incidence of cleft palate which follows steroid administration to laboratory animals does not seem to be echoed in humans, and fetal adrenal suppression seems extremely rare. There is, however, evidence for intrauterine growth retardation where there is prolonged maternal steroid usage. Intravenous beta2-agonists (for instance salbutamol 2.5–5.0 mg four times a day) may be used. Aminophylline is not associated with risk to the fetus, but physicians may have reservations about its safety or usefulness with regard to the mother.

Tetracyclines and, in the third trimester, sulphonamides are contraindicated. Maternal progress should be monitored by repeat blood-gas sampling, and fetal oxygenation by continual fetal monitoring until the acute attack subsides. A baseline pCO_2 of more than 7.1 kPa, or a rise in pCO_2 of more than 1.3 kPa/hr, despite treatment, or maternal exhaustion, are indications for intubation and ventilation. A management plan for status asthmaticus is outlined in Box 10.2.

Box 10.2 The management of status asthmaticus

- Measure blood gases and perform a chest X-ray.
- Commence 100 per cent humidified oxygen.
- Commence IV 5 per cent dextrose.
- Administer nebulized salbutamol or terbutaline and atropine.
- Commence salbutamol or terbutaline infusion.
- Consider aminophylline infusion as per local asthma protocols.
- Commence hydrocortisone infusion 250 mg four times a day.
- Give prednisolone 40 mg orally.
- Commence broad-spectrum antibiotics, for example amoxycillin, if there is consolidation.
- If pCO_2 is more than 7.1 kPa and does not respond rapidly to treatment, or
  if pCO_2 rises more than 1.3 kPa/hr despite treatment, consider intubation and ventilation.

In assessing patients with respiratory tract infection the decrease in functional residual capacity, and the risk to the fetus of pyrexial illness (abortion, intrauterine death, and pre-term labour) should be remembered, and a low threshold for admission should be maintained. Pneumonia is an indication for admission; causative organisms commonly found include *Streptococcus*, *Haemophilus*, and *Klebsiella*. Amoxycillin is a reasonable first-line treatment choice once blood and sputum cultures have been sent.

Patients with chronic lung conditions, such as emphysema

and bronchiectasis, will be adversely affected by the hyperventilation of pregnancy and the effect of the gravid uterus on the muscles of respiration. Assisted delivery may be indicated. Infection should be vigorously treated, and routine antibiotic prophylaxis may be offered. Sarcoidosis improves during pregnancy.

Cardiovascular disease

The increase in cardiac output during pregnancy, the further rise during the second stage of labour, and the sudden increase in blood volume caused by uterine contraction during the third stage all put a significant extra load on the heart. Whilst mild ankle swelling, dyspnoea, and a soft systolic flow murmur may be regarded as normal during pregnancy, diastolic sounds, signs of pulmonary oedema, and dysrhythmias may signify important pathology. Respiratory infection will compound the problem.

If heart failure supervenes, the use of morphine, diuretics, and vasodilators follows standard protocols. During labour, pain-relief must be effective, the second stage short (assistance may be necessary), and other than minimal quantities of intravenous fluids avoided. Epidural anaesthesia is contraindicated, and syntocinon or ergometrine should be avoided in the third stage if possible.

The hormonal changes of pregnancy may affect blood-vessel walls during pregnancy, in that dissecting aortic aneurysms, aortic-valve leaflet rupture, and rupture of splenic artery aneurysms are more common amongst the pregnant than the non-pregnant population.

Neurological disease

Epilepsy may be worsened by pregnancy (45 per cent of patients experience an increased frequency of fitting, 12 per cent a decreased frequency) and drug-handling may be altered; in particular, gastric stasis during labour may lead to a fit through drug non-absorption.

Tonic–clonic seizures during pregnancy may be due to

eclampsia, epilepsy, intracerebral infection, tumour or bleeding, metabolic causes, thrombotic thrombocytopenic purpura, or drug or alcohol (ab)usage. The differential diagnosis is difficult. Patients with epileptic fits may exhibit mild proteinuria due to muscle breakdown and resultant myoglobinuria; their blood pressure may be raised post-ictally. Where the blood pressure is raised a working diagnosis of eclampsia must be made.

During the fit, however, the priorities of management are the same whatever the cause of fitting: the airway must be maintained and safeguarded from aspiration, and the fit must be terminated. A management plan is outlined in Box 10.3.

Box 10.3 **Management of fitting**

- Guard the airway (nurse on the side, head-down; use Guedel airway if tolerated).
- Administer high flow oxygen.
- Give diazepam (as diazemuls) intravenously, 10 mg repeated after 5 minutes. Follow with phenytoin 15–18 mg/kg intravenously over 20–30 minutes. If already on phenytoin reduce dose to 500–1000 mg. Monitor ECG.
- Check blood pressure.
- If the blood pressure is raised treat as eclampsia.
- Check BM stick; if the patient is hypoglycaemic rapidly infuse 1–2 ml/kg of 50 per cent glucose.
- Measure blood glucose, urea, calcium, electrolytes, liver function, clotting, FBC, blood gases; drug screen.
- Screen for anti-convulsant drugs; measure levels urgently if known to be on anti-convulsant medication.
- Check history from relatives, notes, GP *re* possible drug/alcohol abuse.
- Monitor fetus for viability.
- If there is eclampsia refer for delivery.
- If there is not eclampsia refer for urgent CT scan and admission for a neurological opinion.

If the patient is eclamptic, delivery should be effected where there is access to neonatal intensive-care facilities. It is helpful if the emergency physician has sent blood for clotting studies where delivery is judged imminently desirable, as DIC is associated with eclampsia. The fetus should be monitored as soon as the fit is over; an initial bradycardia is not unusual, and is usually self-terminating.

Many patients presenting to emergency departments are poor users of primary care. Epileptics should have their serum drug levels checked to ensure that they remain in the therapeutic range. The importance of such a review of her medication should be stressed to the patient, and referral should be made to obstetric and/ or neurological specialists.

If a patient on phenytoin, primidone, or phenobarbitone presents in labour, the attending physician must ensure that Vitamin K is administered to the neonate.

The hypertrophy of the anterior pituitary gland which accompanies pregnancy may cause compromise of the optic chiasma where there is a pre-existing tumour.

Myasthenia gravis may deteriorate, and neostigmine needs change. Assisted delivery may be needed, and the baby may be hypotonic for the first few days after birth. Exacerbation of disease in the mother is common post-partum.

Gastro-intestinal and hepatic disease

The presentations of appendicitis, cholecystitis, pancreatitis, peptic ulceration, and intestinal obstruction, and the management of these conditions, are discussed in Chapter 9.

Heartburn (gastro-oesophageal reflux) is common in pregnancy, and increases in prevalence (72 per cent in third trimester) and severity with gestational age and parity. Antacids and nocturnal bed-head elevation should be used early, to prevent oesophageal sensitization and severe reflux symptoms.

Jaundice occurring in pregnancy may be due to associated conditions such as oestrogen-induced cholestasis, acute 'fatty liver', toxic hepatitis, and eclampsia, or to coincidental obstructive, infective, and haemolytic causes. Elevated alkaline phosphatase (largely placental) may be mistaken for abnormal liver function in pregnancy. Bilirubin is not raised. However, mild cholestatic jaundice and pruritus accompany pregnancy in women who are unusually sensitive to oestrogens. Resolution occurs when the pregnancy terminates, but there is an increased risk of fetal loss.

'Acute fatty liver' is a rare complication of the third trimester of pregnancy. Fatty degeneration of centrilobar hepatic cells leads to the patient's rapid passage through upper abdominal pain, vomiting, jaundice, clotting deficiency, confusion, and coma to death. This acute condition usually affects young, obese primipara with toxaemia of pregnancy.

During pregnancy there seems to be unusual hepatic sensitivity to chemical agents, and hepatic necrosis may follow the use of halothane, chlorpromazine, and tetracycline.

Infective hepatitis may present with malaise and jaundice, or with non-specific symptoms such as fatigue and nausea, or may be asymptomatic. The mother's progress and management follows the usual course for the non-pregnant patient (cholestyramine resin and prochlorperazine are safe in pregnancy). Hospitalization should be arranged where there is liver failure, coagulopathy, acidosis, or dehydration. Abortion, premature labour and intrauterine death may result. Over 50 per cent of babies born by vaginal delivery to hepatitis B-infected mothers will be B Ag-positive; left untreated, hepatocellular carcinoma or chronic active hepatitis will affect a large percentage of these children. Only 5 per cent of fetuses are infected by transplacental transmission. Caesarean section is therefore the preferred method of delivery, and immunization of the newborn infant should be undertaken shortly after birth. Precautions must be taken to avoid the infection of carers.

Ulcerative colitis may worsen during pregnancy. The acute attack may be treated by standard protocols utilizing prednisolone enemas, oral or intravenous steroid administration, and sulphasalazine, etc. Immunosuppressants such as azathioprine should be avoided.

Endocrine disease

• **Diabetes**   **Adrenal insufficiency**   **Thyroid storm**

Diabetes

Pregnancy is a diabetogenic state. Increased insulin production is accompanied by a decreased sensitivity to insulin. This relative insensitivity is more marked in the obese and the multiparous. Whilst glucose crosses the placenta, insulin cannot; therefore hyperglycaemia in the mother may lead to hypoglycaemia in the fetus due to overproduction of fetal insulin. Lipolysis and ketogenesis are also enhanced by the action of human placental lactogen. The situation is aggravated by raised levels of glucagon, glucocorticoids, catecholamines, and growth hormone. The renal threshold for glucose is lowered, and glycosuria may not reflect a raised blood sugar.

Known diabetics will require increased insulin during pregnancy, and also have a greater tendency to ketosis than normal. Pregnancy-induced hypertension, hydramnios, and preterm labour may accompany diabetes in the mother. Congenital abnormality, intrauterine or neonatal death from hypoglycaemia, intrauterine hypoxia, neonatal respiratory distress syndrome, polycythaemia, neonatal jaundice, hypocalcaemia, and birth trauma due to large fetal size may occur. Maternal retinopathy or nephropathy, or an HbA1c level in excess of 12 per cent are indicators of a poor prognosis. Gestational diabetics may revert to normal after delivery; but a proportion of patients remain diabetic.

During labour, steady control should be ensured by an intravenous glucose and insulin infusion; the fetus must be monitored, and fetal blood sampling must be performed, and the neonate should be transferred to a special care facility for evaluation and treatment if necessary. Diabetic ketoacidosis, whilst contributing little to maternal mortality, is associated with fetal death in more than half the cases. The tendency to ketosis seen in pregnancy leads to significant ketoacidosis at lower blood glucose levels than are normally associated with the condition. The commonest precipitant is infection.

Malaise, headache, nausea, vomiting, polydipsia and poly-uria, and abdominal pain may be amongst the presenting symptoms. The increased plasma volume of later pregnancy may lead to a mismatch between the extent of apparent dehydration and the extent of ketoacidosis, which may disguise the severity of the patient's condition. Box 10.4 contains a management plan for ketoacidosis.

Box 10.4 The management of diabetic ketoacidosis

- Measure blood gases, glucose, urea, and electrolytes.
- Commence intravenous normol saline 1 l in the first hour.
- Give a stat dose of 20 units insulin intravenously.
- Commence an insulin infusion at 6 units/hour.
- Continue fluids at 500–1000 ml/hour for up to four hours, then give 250 ml/hour until urine output is normal and the urine specific gravity is less than 1.02, then maintain at 125 ml/hr.
- Once blood glucose falls below 250 mg/dl change fluid to 5 per cent dextrose. Once normoglycaemic, maintain the patient on an insulin infusion of 1–2 u/hr.
- If potassium level is normal or low initially, give 60 mEq/l infusion. If potassium is initially high give 20 mEq/l in each litre after the first.

Fluid replacement is guided by urine output and specific gravity. Progress should be monitored by repeated checks of blood glucose, electrolyte, and blood-gas levels at one- to two-hourly intervals. Once blood glucose levels have normalized, insulin infusion should be continued at 1 to 2 u/hr until arterial pH and serum bicarbonate levels have also been corrected. As ketones cross the placenta, fetal acidosis will accompany the maternal condition. The fetus should be monitored; but its best chance lies in correction of the mother's condition rather than in premature delivery. Once the mother is stabilized, delivery may be effected for the best management of fetal distress in a neonatal intensive-care facility.

Adrenal insufficiency

A failure to respond to resuscitation after haemorrhage, septicaemia, or amniotic embolism, hypotension during labour or the early puerperium, or collapse associated with the vomiting of early pregnancy may all be due to adrenal insufficiency. Patients with known Addison's disease, or those who have been treated with systemic steroids before or during their pregnancy, should have hydrocortisone 200 mg administered at the onset of labour, and a further 100 mg given each six hours until delivery. Where acute adrenal failure due to haemorrhage into the adrenal glands complicating haemorrhagic or infective shock, or amniotic fluid embolism is suspected, a serum cortisol level should be taken, and 300 mg intravenous hydrocortisone should be administered.

Thyroid disease

The thyroid gland enlarges in pregnancy. Thyroxine-binding globulin, and serum total T4 and T3 are increased. Free T4 is normal or low. Enlargement of a retrosternal simple colloid goitre may cause tracheal compression. Surgery may be performed, and is followed by thyroxine administration. Thyroxine alone will control Hashimoto's thyroiditis. Pregnancy-associated hyperthyroidism is not rare, and is accompanied by fetal hyperthyroidism. It may be disguised by the normal increase in metabolic rate which accompanies pregnancy. A resting tachycardia of more than 100 beats per minute or unexplained weight loss are pointers to overactivity of the gland. Carbimazole or propylthiouracil may be used to control the disease in the mother, but thyroxine should also be given to counteract any resulting fetal hypothyroidism. Radioiodine is contraindicated. Where hyperthyroidism is refractory to medical treatment, partial thyroidectomy may be offered during the middle trimester.

Thyroid storm may accompany labour, pre-eclampsia, severe infection, trauma, operative intervention, or diabetic ketoacidosis. The patient presents with agitation or psychosis, a high temperature, sweating, tachycardia, or supraventricular dysrhythmia, and may progress to cardiac failure, hypotension, and coma. If the clinical picture suggests the diagnosis of thyroid storm (with hyperpyrexia, agitation, tremor, and tachycardia in a patient with known thyroid disease or goitre and exophthalmos), treatment should be commenced without awaiting laboratory free-T4 calculations, as, untreated, the patient may progress through psychosis, dysrhythmia, stupor, coma, and cardiovascular collapse. A management outline is shown in Box 10.5.

Box 10.5 The management of thyroid storm

- Transfer to intensive-care facility and cool the patient.
- Cover infection with broad-spectrum antibiotic.
- Generous intravenous fluid replacement.
- Propranolol 1–2 mg/minute IV up to 10 mg.
- Propylthiouracil 300 to 600 mg orally or by nasogastric tube.
- Potassium iodide orally or via NGT, 5 drops.
- Hydrocortisone 100 mg IV.
- Continue propranolol 40–80 mg, propylthiouracil 150–300 mg, and potassium iodide 5 drops, 6-hourly and hydrocortisone 100 mg 8-hourly.

Parenteral steroids are prescribed, as ACTH secretion is thought to be inadequate during a thyroid crisis.

Myxoedemic patients have an increased requirement for thyroxine during pregnancy.

Haemoglobinopathies and anaemia

No woman should commence labour with a haemoglobin level below 10 g/dl. Most cases of iron or folate deficiency are recognized and treated in the antenatal clinic. However, women with poor social conditions and those from tropical countries are both the most at risk of profound anaemia and the most likely to present to the emergency department in labour. Blood transfusion is the only rapid way of raising the haemoglobin level. Unless there is a history of recent haemorrhage, this is safest given as packed cells, with diuretic cover. Exchange transfusion may be indicated for very profound anaemias (Hb 5 g/dl or less) or where there is cardiac failure.

Haemoglobin S is the name given to a haemoglobin molecule when the glutamic acid at position 6 in the β-chain of the normal adult haemoglobin (haemoglobin A) is replaced by valine. Where this haemoglobin is inherited from both parents (sickle-cell anaemia), the red cells take on a sickle shape when oxygen tension is low, clump together, blocking vessels in the micro-circulation, and cause infarction. Pregnancy may be accompanied by hypertension and sickle-cell crises. Painful crises are the most common; the precipitating factor (for instance infection) should be sought, and the crisis treated with intravenous fluids (60 ml/kg/24 hrs), oxygen, and analgesia (intravenous opioid infusion, for example pethidine 0.5 mg/kg/hr adjusted as necessary to control pain). Full blood count, urea and electrolytes, liver-function tests, blood cultures, and chest X-ray should be taken. Lung crisis, where intrapulmonary sickling mimics pulmonary embolism/infection, is the major cause of death for a sickling patient. Coronary or cerebral thrombosis may occur. The placental vessels may thrombose, causing fetal death, and there is commonly intrauterine growth retardation. There is an increased incidence of abortion and preterm labour. The heterozygous state (sickle-cell trait) is usually well tolerated in pregnancy, although there is a tendency to pyelonephritis.

Haemoglobin C is caused by the replacement of the glutamic acid with lysine. The rare homozygous HbC anaemia causes a mild haemolytic anaemia. The combination of haemoglobins S and C presents a similar clinical picture to haemoglobin SS disease.

Thalassaemia is caused by impaired production of either the α or β chains of haemoglobin. Two α thalassaemia trait parents may give rise to the disease in the fetus, which is hydropic and dies soon after birth. There is a risk of severe pre-eclampsia, and obstructed labour in the mother. Mothers who have α trait have varying degrees of microcytic, hypochromic anaemia. Pregnancy in β thalassaemia major sufferers is very rare; the minor form causes a mild microcytic anaemia. Where there is a possibility of significant haemolysis daily folate supplements of 5 mg/day should be given throughout pregnancy. Iron-deficiency anaemia should have been excluded.

Dermatological conditions

Herpes gestationis is a rare complication of pregnancy, but may lead to severe illness, and even death, in the mother and to abortion and the intrauterine death of the fetus. The patient experiences severe pruritus, followed by erythematous patches on the abdomen and legs which progress to crops of vesicles and haemorrhagic and pustular bullae. There is systemic illness, with pyrexia, rigors, and vomiting. A high eosinophil count is found. Treatment consists of intravenous steroids and antibiotics as indicated.

Communicable disease

The patient with a high pyrexia may lose her child from abortion, intrauterine death, or pre-term labour.

Septic shock from whatever cause is a dire emergency for mother and child. The patient presents with any of the clinical signs and symptoms summarized in Box 10.6.

A careful history must be taken to identify the likely origin of the infection. Blood and urine cultures, swabs, and a chest X-ray are taken. An ECG and tests of renal and hepatic function and clotting studies should be performed. Unless otherwise guided, treatment is commenced immediately on the assumption the parent infection is pelvic with a broad-spectrum combination, for example cefotaxime/ metronidazole. DIC should be actively sought and promptly treated.

Box 10.6 **Signs and symptoms of septicaemic shock**

- There is hypotension, with either flushed or cold peripheries.
- There may be the signs and symptoms of a localized infection, for example of a wound or kidney.
- Disseminated intravascular coagulopathy may supervene, with bleeding from puncture sites and haemorrhage.

Cerebral
- Confusion
- Labile temperature control

Cardiac
- Tachycardia
- Dysrhythmia
- Heart failure
- Infarction

Respiratory
- Tachypnoea, dyspnoea
- Pulmonary oedema
- Haemorrhage
- ARDS

Renal
- Failure
- Haematuria

Hepatic
- Enlargement
- Jaundice
- Failure

Gastro-intestinal
- Ileus
- Vomiting

In addition to these general risks there are specific dangers to mother or child associated with certain infections.

Infection with measles or chickenpox may spread to the fetus, and the child may be born with a rash; rarely, congenital abnormalities follow chickenpox. Influenza in the first trimester may lead to a small rise in congenital abnormalities. There is an increased susceptibility to polio and Sydenham's chorea during pregnancy. Infection of the mother with rubella, toxoplasmosis, and cytomegalic virus may lead to multiple congenital abnormalities or intra-uterine or infant death. Whenever there is a clinical suspicion of rubella, antibody testing should be performed and the patient referred for follow-up. The patient should be kept well away from other pregnant women during the course of her infection. An antibody test is also available for toxoplasmosis.

Around 2000 women are thought to be infected with HIV in the UK. Estimates of the level of HIV infection amongst women attending antenatal clinics vary, one study giving a prevalence of 10 cases per 3500 attenders.

The coexistence of other sexually transmitted infections, particularly those causing ulceration of the genitalia, increases the risk of infection. Transmission is more common in early or end-stage infection. The average time between HIV infection and the onset of AIDS is seven years. Viral antigen can be found in blood a few weeks after infection; although the appearance of antibody may take up to a year, 90 per cent of patients are seroconverted by six months, and most tests are positive within three months of infection. False negatives may also be found in very advanced disease. False positives may occur, and the patient should be retested before any verdict is passed.

HIV infection may increase the risk of cervical neoplasia, sexually transmitted disease, genital herpes, and pelvic tuberculosis. Infection of the fetus *in utero* is well documented. The estimation of risk varies from 15–51 per cent, and is thought to be lower when the mother is clinically well. There may be an increased risk of preterm labour where the mother is symptomatic. Most HIV-antibody screening kits detect IgG. The first antigen-specific antibodies produced by infants are usually IgM. Maternal IgG crosses the placenta, and may persist for up to 15 months. A positive test in a neonate is therefore of no predictive value, and follow-up testing over the first two years of life is indicated, the mean age of diagnosis of vertically infected children being 2 years 4 months. Clinically, signs of infection in the infant include hepato-splenomegaly, lymphadenopathy, and microcephaly. The HIV virus has been found in breast milk, and breast-feeding is not recommended in this country.

There is some evidence that acceleration of the progress of AIDS may accompany pregnancy and birth; this appears to be true only of symptomatic mothers.

The emergency physician must now take routine precautions against HIV infection whenever body fluids are handled. Gloves should be routinely worn when delivering a baby.

The HIV virus withstands drying at room temperature, but is killed by pH less than 2 or more than 13, by heating to 56 degrees for 30 minutes, or by hypochlorite, glutaraldehyde, and lipid solvents. A 1:10 solution of sodium hypochlorite may be used to clean body-fluid spillage. When the mother is known to be HIV-positive or to be an intravenous drug-abuser, the infection risk should be minimized by delivery in a side-ward, and the use of gowns, goggles, masks, and gloves. Disposable items should be used as much as possible, and the labour area and instruments should be cleaned after delivery with 1:10 sodium hypochlorite solution. All soiled linen or clinical waste, specimens from the patient, and the placenta should be 'double-bagged' and labelled with biological hazard stickers. Mouth-operated suction devices should not be used. Gloves should be worn when handling the newborn infant's cord, or dealing with urine, faeces, or vomit. Disposable nappies are recommended.

Listeriosis presents with any degree of illness from asymptomatic carriage to septicaemia and death. Commonly, the mother experiences a mild flu-like illness, with fever, headache, muscle and back pain, and, sometimes, gastrointestinal symptoms. The patient may be misdiagnosed as suffering from pyelonephritis. Infection of the fetus may result in mid-trimester abortion, stillbirth, or premature birth. Examination of the mother yields no specific findings. Any pregnant woman with a non-specific pyrexia of over 38 degrees which has persisted for 48 hours, must be treated as possibly infected with *Listeria*. A blood culture should be sent and the patient should be started immediately on high-dose ampicillin (or erythromycin if she is allergic to penicillin). Any pregnant woman presenting with an early pyrexia of unknown origin must be watched carefully: persistence to 48 hours should be treated as above.

Malarial infection not uncommonly presents to emergency medicine departments. The pregnant patient has an increased susceptibility to the disease, and pregnancy both exacerbates the acute attack and may lead to the recrudescence of latent disease. Abortion, intrauterine growth retardation, and pre-term labour are common. Malarial parasites will usually be demonstrated on a thick blood film. The patient should be admitted. Chloroquine is the treatment of choice. Where the patient is from a chloroquine-resistant zone, the combination of pyrimethamine and dapsone is recommended. In all cases the advice of the Public Health Laboratory should be sought.

Giardiasis may present with offensive diarrhoea, vomiting, and fatigue. Malabsorption and dehydration may ensue. The diagnosis is made by examination of a fresh stool specimen, and treatment, if indicated by the state of the patient, uses metronidazole 200 mg three times a day for five days. Metronidazole, however, is contraindicated in the first trimester and when breast-feeding.

Gastro-enteritis is usually self-limiting, the danger to mother and fetus lying in the risk of dehydration. If the mother is unwell, is pyrexial, is passing stools in excess of 10/day or blood with the stool, or is clinically dehydrating admission and possible intravenous rehydration are indicated.

The management of infective vaginitis or primary syphilis is described in Chapter 4, that of herpetic infection in Chapter 3.

Dependency

Although pregnancy is not common in the chronic opiate addict, female street addicts are more likely to bring their obstetric problems to the emergency department than to the antenatal clinic. They may also present in advanced labour. As well as risking hepatitis and HIV infection, such women are malnourished, and prone to systemic, localized, and sexually transmitted infection. The effects on the fetus include intrauterine growth retardation, premature birth, and neonatal drug-withdrawal symptoms. If the baby sneezes within the first few hours of birth, withdrawal symptoms are starting. Oral chlorpromazine should be given to the infant immediately. If the mother wishes to discharge herself and her child, child-protection procedures should be initiated and the child should be admitted under the care of the paediatric and social services.

Alcoholic mothers may also present. The fetus is likely to be small and may have the fetal alcohol syndrome. Perinatal mortality rates are raised.

Psychiatric disease

The incidence and aetiology of psychiatric disease are probably the same in pregnant women as those amongst the comparable non-pregnant population. Pregnancy has no specific effect on psychotic disease, although the anticipation of labour, and worries about coping with the child, may adversely affect anxiety-based conditions.

Any mother bringing a child where there is a suspicion of abuse, or expressing an inappropriate level of anxiety about her child's condition, must be assessed for possible psychiatric illness.

The main difficulties for the emergency physician accompany the urgent control of a psychiatric crisis; and the emergency department also has a role to play in the revision of drug therapy commenced before the pregnancy was known.

Lithium must be avoided at all stages of pregnancy. The discontinuation of lithium therapy may lead to difficulties in controlling manic depression, and this group of patients may present acutely disturbed in the first trimester.

Benzodiazepines are contraindicated in the third trimester, and probably better avoided throughout gestation.

Antidepressants and antipsychotic medications, by contrast, are generally safe, although occasional adverse effects on the neonate have been reported (extrapyramidal reactions with antipsychotics and hyperarousal phenomena with antidepressants), and they are best avoided if possible in the third trimester.

Electroconvulsive therapy appears to be unattended by adverse effects on the fetus.

The emergency physician faced with an acutely psychotic patient should therefore consider therapy in line with usual departmental protocols. Haloperidol 10–30 mg IM or chlorpromazine 25–50 mg IM are reasonable first choices.

Further reading

Calman, K. C. (1992). Management and prevention of listeriosis and other food-borne infections in pregnancy, PL/CMO (92)19. Department of Health, London.

De Swiet, M. (ed.) (1989). *Medical disorders in obstetric practice* (2nd edn.). Blackwell Scientific Publications, Oxford.

HIV infection in obstetrics and gynaecology (1992). *Baillière's clinical obstetrics and gynaecology*, **6**(1), 1–216.

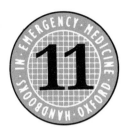

CHAPTER 11

The pregnant patient presenting with injury

Key points in the pregnant patient presenting with injury

1 The assessment and resuscitation of the injured mother are importantly altered by the changes in respiratory and cardiovascular function which accompany pregnancy.

2 High-flow oxygen must be routinely administered to any pregnant woman with other than a trivial limb injury.

3 The pregnant patient can lose 35 per cent of her blood volume before manifesting any of the classical signs and symptoms of shock. Vigorous fluid infusion and early blood transfusion are required to avoid the attendant severe fetal compromise.

4 Supine hypotension which results from compression of the inferior vena cava by the gravid uterus must be avoided by nursing the patient on her left side or by elevating the right buttock and displacing the uterus to the left manually.

5 The assessment of abdominal haemorrhage is difficult in the pregnant patient; computed tomography is the investigation of choice but diagnostic peritoneal lavage, inserting the cannula just cranial to the fundus in the midline, may be used.

6 The fetal outlook is primarily dependent on the mother's resuscitation and recovery.

7 The second greatest threat to fetal survival is abruption of the placenta. The mother's transfusion needs must be immediately revised if bleeding *per vaginam* or uterine tenderness are present.

Injury to the mother

Boxes 11.1 and 11.2 serve as a reminder of the physiological changes which accompany pregnancy and may alter the expression of injury. In addition the mass effect of the uterus alters the pattern of injury. Box 11.3 summarizes these changes.

The primary survey* of the injured mother and her initial resuscitation are altered in certain significant aspects by these changes.

Box 11.1 Physiological changes of pregnancy relevant to trauma

- Blood volume up 50 per cent
- Red cell mass up 25 per cent
- Cardiac output up 30 per cent
- CVP down 60 per cent (supine)
- Supine hypotension (cardiac output falls by up to 30 per cent, CVP by up to 66 per cent).
- Peripheral resistance down
- Paradoxical vasodilatation in response to shock (1st and 2nd trimesters)
- Mean arterial pressure fall of 5–15 mmHg (second trimester)
- Pulse rate up 20 bpm
- Third heart sound and systolic murmur
- L axis on ECG, inverted T waves in 111, V1, and V2
- Decreased functional residual capacity
- Tidal volume 40 per cent increased
- Relaxed lower oesophageal sphincter
- Slow gastric emptying, decreased gastro-intestinal motility
- Renal plasma flow up
- Enlargement of pituitary gland

---

* As defined by the ATLS protocol of the American College of Surgeons.

Box 11.2 **Laboratory data norms in pregnancy**
- Haematocrit 32–41 per cent
- Haemoglobin 11–15 g/100 ml
- White cell count 5000–16 000/mm^3 but may rise as high as 25 000 under stress, for example labour
- Platelets 134 000–400 000/mm^3
- ESR 44–114 mm/hr
- Fibrinogen 4–6 g/100 ml
- Fibrin degradation products 14.0 ± 7.0
- pCO_2 27–32 mmHg
- pO_2 100–108 mmHg
- HCO_3 18–23 mmol
- Creatinine 38–90 µmol/l
- Urea 1.6–6.0 mmol/l
- Albumen 28–40 g/l
- Alkaline phosphatase rises through pregnancy: first trimester 33–87 iu/l, second trimester 31–117 iu/l, third trimester 69–209 iu/l

Box 11.3 **Organs at increased risk of injury during pregnancy**
- Spleen
- Bladder
- Small bowel in upper abdominal trauma
- Pelvic vessels
- Lung:—Increased risk of thromboembolism
        —Lung atelectasis
        —Aspiration of gastric contents

Organs at decreased risk of injury during pregnancy
- Pelvic fracture
- Bowel may be shielded

The decrease in functional residual capacity is normally compensated by the 'hyperventilation of pregnancy' under the stimulus of progesterone, with the increased tidal and minute volumes causing lowering of the pCO_2, which is balanced by a fall in serum bicarbonate. When hypoventilation occurs oxygenation is very vulnerable. Prompt management of the airway and thoracic injury are particularly important. Chest drains should be inserted one or two intercostal spaces above the usual site. If assisted ventilation is required the patient should be hyperventilated to simulate the normal adaptation.

In addition the shift to the left of the oxygen dissociation curve characteristic of fetal haemoglobin means that when maternal haemoglobin is fully saturated, fetal haemoglobin is only two-thirds saturated, and the fetus will continue to benefit from oxygen given to the mother. High-flow oxygen should be routinely administered to any pregnant woman with other than minor extremity injury pending further evaluation. The relaxation of the gastro-oesophageal sphincter and the decrease in gastric emptying encourage gastro-oesophageal reflux. The lungs should be protected from the risk of aspiration by the insertion of a nasogastric tube.

The vasodilatation which is noted in pregnancy, the hampering of venous return by the gravid uterus, and the paradoxical vasodilatation in response to shock which is seen in the first two trimesters, all make the maternal circulation lack the efficient peripheral vasoconstriction which is part of the normal response to blood loss. In addition the massive expansion of the blood volume gives a cushioning effect to the maternal expression of hypovolaemia. This cushion does not extend to the fetus. The uteroplacental circulation rapidly contracts. The pregnant patient can, as a result of the disguise these physiological changes provide, lose 35 per cent of her blood volume before manifesting any of the 'classical' signs and symptoms of shock. To avoid the attendant severe fetal compromise, fluid resuscitation of the pregnant patient should be vigorous, and blood transfusion will be necessary early in management to safeguard fetal oxygenation. In monitoring fluid needs the baseline CVP is variable, but its response to infusion parallels that seen in non-pregnant patients. Vasopressors should be avoided, as they further decrease the uterine circulation. There is a risk of disseminated intravascular coagulopathy supervening, and clotting studies should be taken with the baseline blood tests and repeated.

'Supine hypotension' must be avoided, either by nursing the patient on her left side or, where that is contraindicated, by elevating the right buttock and displacing the uterus to the left manually. When the patient is immobilized on a spinal board the board may be elevated on the right giving a tilt of some fifteen to twenty degrees.

. The main part of the **secondary survey*** follows standard guidelines, with the addition of an evaluation of the uterus and fetus. The possibility that fitting or coma may be due to eclampsia rather than head injury must be remembered. The 'classical' signs of hypertension, hyperreflexia, oedema, and proteinuria are not always present.

Whilst the relaxation of the symphysis pubis and sacroiliac joints make pelvic fracture less likely than in the non-pregnant state, the increased vascular supply to the pelvic area means that intra- or retro-peritoneal bleeding may be catastrophic. The veins of the broad ligament may be damaged by blunt or penetrating trauma, giving rise to a haematoma which may require bilateral internal iliac and ovarian vessel ligation to control. Uterine damage that involves the uterine vessels requires immediate Caesarean section for both fetal and maternal stabilization.

The spleen is injured more commonly in later pregnancy than is usual, and such injury is associated with a 15 per cent mortality, contributed to by a failure of diagnosis. The assessment of abdominal haemorrhage may be difficult when the patient is pregnant because of the interposition of the uterus between the examiner and the examined structures, and also because of the damping of signs of peritonism by the stretched abdominal wall. Retroperitoneal haemorrhage is best diagnosed by computed tomography (CT), which will also indicate intraperitoneal haemorrhage, and, sometimes, the area of damage responsible. Where the patient's state, or the available facilities, preclude the use of CT, diagnostic peritoneal lavage should be performed where there are uncertain abdominal signs, the patient is obtunded, general anaesthesia is planned imminently, or continuing hypotension suggests intra-abdominal blood loss. The open tech-

* As defined by the ATLS protocol of the American College of Surgeons.

nique is used, the site of entry being just cranial to the uterine fundus in the midline. The usual criteria of the aspiration of more than 5 ml of fresh blood or bowel contents, the passage of lavage fluid into chest drain or urinary catheter, or the finding of more than 100 000 red blood cells/mm^3 or more than 500 white cells/mm^3 in the lavage fluid, are used as indicators for laparotomy.

Laboratory investigations should include group and cross-match, full blood count, biochemistry, urinalysis, and clotting studies. The last should be routinely performed because of the association of abruptio placentae with disseminated intravascular coagulation.

The indications for surgery, use of tetanus prophylaxis, and antibiotic cover remain the same as for the non-pregnant patient. Tetracycline, chloramphenicol, and sulphonamides should be avoided. Caesarean section should only be performed for the usual obstetric reasons unless it is needed for exposure of the surgical field or fetal distress.

Injury to the uterus and fetus

The fetal outlook is predominantly dependent on the mother's resuscitation and recovery. Maternal hypotension is correlated with a poor outcome (80 per cent fetal mortality).

In the first trimester, the uterus is protected by the bony pelvis, and there is no well-validated evidence of fetal loss due to trauma in this group. As pregnancy progresses, the uterus rises above the pelvic brim and becomes increasingly thin-walled, the fetus is less cushioned by amniotic fluid, and the head becomes fixed in the pelvic brim (engaged) by term. It therefore becomes steadily more vulnerable to both direct and indirect trauma. Lap seat-belts have been implicated in uterine trauma received during road-traffic accidents.

A rough estimate of the length of gestation is made by assessing the uterine fundal height (see Fig. 1.1, p. 9): from 20 weeks' gestation the age of the fetus in weeks approximates to the distance from symphysis to pubis in centimetres. Once this reaches 24 weeks, the fetus must be regarded as potentially viable.

The fundal height should be marked on the abdominal wall as a guide to any increase in uterine size (an indicator of placental abruption). The uterus is examined for tenderness and irritability. Labour pains are characteristically bilateral, generalized, last at least 40 seconds, and become regularly spaced at less than eight-minute intervals before cervical effacement and dilatation begin. By contrast, constant or irregular abdominal pain or backache, localized tenderness, and vaginal bleeding are indicators of uterine trauma or placental abruption. Should preterm labour commence, the first approach is to correct hypovolaemia and hypoxia and to assess the patient for uterine injury, abruption, or intra-peritoneal bleeding. Tocolytics should be withheld altogether unless there is progressive cervical change. Ritodrine should be used with extreme caution, as its side-effects may have a serious adverse effect on the unstable patient.

No tocolytic agent will work once cervical dilatation has reached 4 cm, or if the membranes are ruptured.

A pelvic examination should be made as part of the routine assessment of the patient. Where there is bleeding or fluid leakage per vaginam and the mother is more than 20 weeks pregnant, the examination is best performed by an obstetrician. A sterile speculum should be used, avoiding the risk of introducing infection or disrupting a placenta praevia by digital examination. If there is evidence of rupture of the membranes (amniotic fluid has a pH of 7.4–7.5), cervical cultures should be taken for Chlamydia, Gonococcus, and Streptococcus. Amniotic fluid may also be found on peritoneal lavage after penetrating injury to the uterus.

The fetus should be monitored continuously. Where the degree of abdominal trauma is mild a few hours' observation will suffice; where trauma is more severe, monitoring should be continued for at least 48 hours. Potentially lethal abruptio placentae should become clinically evident within this period, although milder degrees may take up to 5 days to present. If the cardiotocograph shows an abnormal fetal heart rate, the fetus should be delivered promptly by Caesarean section. The greatest threat to fetal survival being inadequate resuscitation of the mother, the second greatest is **abruption of the placenta**. Fetal death rates from placental abruption have been quoted to be as high as 60 per cent, with estimates of abruption in severely injured mothers ranging from 6 to 66 per cent. The presentation and management of abruption is similar to that of non-traumatic origin.

Three features of the condition are particularly relevant to the management of trauma. As a significant portion of the haemorrhage associated with abruption is 'concealed', and therefore blood loss may be dangerously underestimated, the mother's transfusion needs must be immediately revised if bleeding *per vaginam* or uterine tenderness are present. Secondly, abruption is a cause of disseminated intravascular coagulation, which must be sought by clotting studies and careful observation of the patient. Most cases present within six hours of trauma, and may therefore become evident in the Emergency Department. Thirdly, fetomaternal haemorrhage may ensue, causing fetal anaemia, anoxia, or death. Evidence that haemorrhage has occurred is afforded by the Betke–Kleihauer test, which detects fetal red blood cells; the proportion of fetal to maternal cells can be used to estimate the extent of blood loss. If the mother is Rhesus-negative, anti-D immunoglobulin should be given, however slight the haemorrhage.

Uterine rupture is less common than placental abruption (estimated at about 1 per cent of severely injured pregnant women). A small tear may present only an area of uterine tenderness. A major rupture will be accompanied by haemorrhagic shock. The fetal parts may be unusually easily palpated, and abnormally positioned. The uterus may be palpable as a separate firm mass; X-ray may show a pneumoperitoneum; and peritoneal lavage returns blood and amniotic fluid. Immediate laparotomy is indicated with any degree of tear. Repair without disturbing the fetus may be possible with small tears; otherwise the uterus is emptied and repaired, unless the degree of bleeding demands a hysterectomy.

Direct injury to the fetus from blunt trauma is rare, the most common being skull fracture and intracranial haemorrhage. Extremely rarely, placental or cord damage may be found, often out of proportion to the severity of maternal injury.

Amniotic fluid embolism may be a rare consequence of

trauma. The patient suffers sudden dyspnoea, hypotension, cyanosis, haemorrhage, and fitting. Coma and death rapidly supervene in half the cases. Survivors of the first few minutes develop disseminated intravascular coagulation, and require treatment of this condition together with inotropic support and ventilation as required.

Penetrating injury to the abdomen may result from stab wounds of the abdomen. Unless peritoneal lavage suggests severe bleeding from the uterine wound, or there is fetal distress, an expectant policy may be adopted for lower abdominal injuries once a cystogram has ruled out bladder injury. Laparotomy will be needed for upper abdominal wounds, given the greater likelihood of visceral injury; but again the aim of surgery is to be as conservative as possible.

Gunshot wounds to the abdomen are associated with a poor fetal prognosis (40–70 per cent die, 60–90 per cent are injured), whilst maternal morbidity and mortality are low. Laparotomy is mandatory. Where the uterus is uninjured, the pregnancy should be left intact. Where there is injury, the fetus of more than 34 weeks' gestation should be delivered. At earlier dates than this the fetus is as likely to die from prematurity as from its wounds. The trend is therefore towards conservative management.

Further reading

Robertson, C. and Redmond, A. D. (1991). *The management of major trauma*, Oxford Handbooks in Emergency Medicine. Oxford University Press.

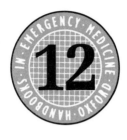

CHAPTER 12

The patient with a systemic complication of pregnancy

Key points in the patient with a systemic complication of pregnancy

1 If vomiting in pregnancy becomes severe or persistent, intercurrent illness must first be considered and discounted (particularly pyelonephritis and intestinal obstruction) before the diagnosis of hyperemesis gravidarum is made.

2 Half the cases of deep venous thrombosis in pregnant women are asymptomatic. The maternal mortality of untreated embolism is 13 per cent. Any pregnant woman presenting with dyspnoea or chest pain must be immediately assessed with the possibility of a pulmonary embolism in mind.

3 Abruptio placentae, intra-uterine death, and missed abortion are the most common obstetric causes of disseminated intravascular coagulation. Careful watch must be kept for the combination of microvascular thrombosis and haemorrhage which characterize this condition.

4 Hypertension during pregnancy is assessed relative to the individual patient's norm, an increase of 15 mmHg diastolic pressure over the patient's pre-pregnant or early trimester level, being taken as significant. A blood pressure over 140/90 is routinely regarded as abnormal and a level above 110 mmHg diastolic is regarded as severe.

5 Pre-eclampsia may be defined as the manifestation of a utero-placental disorder causing widespread systemic disturbance in the mother. In some cases the mother presents primarily with liver damage, thrombocytopenia, and microangiopathic haemolysis without the conventional markers of pre-eclampsia—the HELLP syndrome. Eclampsia may be defined as the onset of fitting after the 20th week of gestation.

6 All pregnant women with a blood pressure above 140/90 should be referred to the duty obstetrician for consideration of admission. Extreme pre-eclampsia may need the commencement of treatment in the emergency department. Eclamptic fitting must be promptly controlled by intravenous diazepam, chlormethiazole, or phenytoin as necessary.

Hyperemesis gravidarum

Nausea and vomiting are very common features of the early weeks of pregnancy. It is unusual for symptoms to persist beyond the 14th week, and the mother remains well in herself. Women attend the emergency department who are complaining of vomiting which they feel to be excessive but who are objectively well. Cyclizine and promethazine are safe antiemetics to use in pregnancy, and can be used to supplement the reassurance which should be offered. If the vomiting becomes severe or persistent, intercurrent illness must first be considered and discounted, particularly pyelonephritis and intestinal obstruction.

Hyperemesis gravidarum is defined as the persistence of pregnancy-related vomiting to the degree that it affects the mother's health. The patient dehydrates, and oliguria, tachycardia, hypotension, and weight loss may occur. In addition vitamin deficiency is a risk, and hepatic necrosis has been reported. Laboratory testing reveals electrolyte imbalance, a raised urea, and ketosis. About a third of sufferers show transient hyperthyroxinaemia, possibly due to a stimulant effect of HCG, or a variant of HCG, on the thyroid gland. The sufferer from the full-blown picture must be admitted for rehydration, and an intravenous infusion should be commenced.

Deep venous thrombosis (DVT)

Estimates of the incidence of **deep venous thrombosis** during pregnancy range from 0.3 to 12.0 per 1000: 66 per cent postpartum, the time-scale for presentation varying from two days to four weeks; 25 per cent embolize to the lungs. The tendency to thrombose is made up of the elements of changed blood composition (increased fibrinogen and factors II, VII, VIII, IX, and X, and decreased plasminogen activator) giving a hypercoaguable state, slowed flow from inferior vena caval compression by the uterus (flow is reduced by 50 per cent by the third trimester), venous dilatation, immobility, peroperative pressure on the legs, and vessel-wall damage from instrumentation or sepsis. The aetiology is summarized in Box 12.1.

Box 12.1 Aetiology of thromboembolism

- Caesarean section
- general anaesthesia
- instrumentation
- high parity
- advanced maternal age
- poor social circumstances and nutrition
- more common in A, B, or AB blood groups
- obesity
- decreased mobility, for instance in bedrest for pre-eclampsia
- previous deep venous thrombosis (recurrence rate 12:100)
- varicose veins
- cardiovascular disease
- SLE
- AT3 deficiency
- sickle-cell disease
- trauma and traumatic delivery
- infection
- haemoconcentration, for example dehydration, polycythaemia, hypotension
- carcinoma

Half the cases of DVT are asymptomatic. Of those with the classic signs of oedema, calf tenderness and Homan's sign, half do not have DVT. Ultrasound examination should reveal a clot, and is preferred to venography.

Pulmonary embolism (PE)

Pulmonary embolism may present with cardiovascular collapse or shortness of breath, chest pain, cough, syncope, or haemoptysis. There may be tachypnoea, hypotension, tachycardia, pyrexia, cyanosis, raised central venous pressure, a pleural rub, and the signs of a pulmonary effusion. A feeling of impending catastrophe is sometimes described by the patient. Diagnosis may be difficult, but the maternal mortality of untreated embolism is 13 per cent. Any pregnant woman presenting with dyspnoea or chest pain must be immediately assessed with the possibility of a pulmonary embolism in mind. The electrocardiogram shows T wave inversion in 40 per cent, and a right-axis shift if the embolus is large. In 90 per cent of patients the paO_2 falls below 80. Whilst hypocarbia is normal in pregnancy, hypoxia never is.

The need to be certain of the diagnosis dictates that appropriate investigations must be carried out (perfusion or ventilation–perfusion lung scan).

Treatment of DVT or PE must be commenced in the emergency department. Thrombolysis, embolectomy, and IVC intervention are reserved for mothers *in extremis*. Warfarin is contraindicated in pregnancy, but heparin may be safely used, as it does not cross the placenta. An initial loading dose of 70 u/kg is followed by infusion of 1000 u or more per hour, depending on the APTT, which should be measured four-hourly. This is continued as an inpatient for seven to ten days, and then followed by a regime of subcutaneous heparin, aimed at keeping the APTT about 1.5 times the control until delivery. Warfarin may be commenced after delivery, and is continued for three to six months.

Disseminated intravascular coagulation (DIC)

Disseminated intravascular coagulation is a condition of abnormal coagulation and fibrinolysis. Thromboplastins are released into the circulation from placental or decidual tissue, activating the clotting cascade intravascularly, consuming clotting factors, and depositing fibrin. The fibrinolytic cascade is activated in response, generating fibrin degradation products. The consumption of coagulation factors and anticoagulant properties of FDPs causes a haemorrhagic state. The clinical picture is caused by this combination of widespread microvascular occlusion and haemorrhage. Endothelial cell injury may be the initiator in sepsis and eclampsia. Phospholipids from blood-cell injury may be the mechanism in transfusion. The aetiological factors are summarized in Box 12.2, the league leaders being abruptio, intrauterine death, and missed abortion.

Box 12.2 **Aetiology of DIC (obstetric causes only)**

- abruptio placentae
- intrauterine death
- missed abortion
- amniotic fluid embolism
- uterine rupture
- eclampsia
- massive transfusion
- sepsis
- trophoblastic disease
- saline abortion

The clinical picture of the cause is accompanied by signs such as bruising, purpura, or venepuncture site or wound oozing, or by frank post-partum haemorrhage. Multisystem dysfunction is caused by the thrombotic manifestations.

Clotting studies show long prothrombin and thrombin times, high levels of FDPs, and falling fibrinogen levels and platelet counts. Microangiopathic haemolytic anaemia may ensue.

Treatment has three elements: maintaining the supply of oxygen to the tissues, replacing coagulation factors, and removing the cause. Oxygen is administered and the intravascular volume rapidly restored with a colloid or crystalloid solution initially, followed by bank red cells and fresh frozen plasma as soon as the blood is cross-matched. Progress should be carefully monitored, including urine output and CVP. Once hypovolaemia is corrected delivery should be expedited.

Pre-eclampsia and eclampsia

Pre-eclampsia is traditionally defined as the onset of hypertension, proteinuria, and oedema after the 20th week of pregnancy. It complicates 7 per cent of pregnancies. **Eclampsia** is traditionally defined by the addition of fits to the above. Modern obstetric management has reduced the incidence of eclampsia to less than 0.1 per cent. Eclampsia occurs ante-partum in 50 per cent of cases, intra-partum in 25 per cent, and post-partum in 25 per cent (66 per cent of which present more than 48 hours after birth). There may be no history of ante-partum pre-eclampsia in those who present with eclampsia post-partum.

Pre-eclampsia is better defined as the manifestation of a utero-placental disorder causing widespread systemic disturbance in the mother, including the renal, cardiovascular, coagulation, and hepatic systems (see Box 12.3).

Box 12.3 **Manifestations of pre-eclampsia/eclampsia**

Renal
- Glomerular endotheliosis
- Impaired tubular and glomerular function
- Hyperuricaemia
- Proteinuria
- Acute renal failure with tubular or cortical necrosis
- Hypoalbuminaemia and sodium/potassium retention contributing to oedema

Cardiovascular
- Hypertension (increased peripheral resistance, variable change in cardiac output)
- Hypovolaemia
- Arterial injury
- Cardiac necrosis and haemorrhage

Haematological
- Thrombocytopenia
- Abnormal platelets

- Abnormalities of clotting-factor turnover
- Disseminated intravascular coagulopathy
- Microangiopathic anaemia

Hepatic
- Abnormal liver enzymes
- Periportal haemorrhage
- Portal tract thromboses
- Infarction
- Rupture

Neurological
- Convulsions
- Intracerebral haemorrhage
- Intracerebral oedema
- Intracerebral infarct
- Retinal oedema and detachment

Respiratory
- Pulmonary oedema
- Laryngeal oedema
- Haemorrhage

Placental/Fetal
- Placental infarction
- Abruptio placentæ
- Fetal intrauterine growth retardation
- Fetal death

Eclampsia is better defined as the onset of fitting after the 20th week of gestation, as 20 per cent of cases have no proteinuria and 40 per cent no oedema. The causation of pre-eclampsia is uncertain; there is evidence that there is an imbalance in the production of thromboxane A2 and prostacyclin, with thromboxane being relatively high. There is generalized vasoconstriction, accompanied by intravascular fibrin deposition and platelet adherence with thrombocytopenia in some cases.

The aetiology is summarized in Box 12.4.

Box 12.4 **Aetiology of pre-eclampsia/eclampsia**

• Primigravidae
• Age less than 20 or more than 35
• Poor social circumstances and nutrition
• Multiple pregnancy
• Familial
• Gestational trophoblastic disease
• Polyhydramnios
• Hydrops fetalis
• Abdominal pregnancy
• Diabetes mellitus
• Chronic hypertension
• Collagen vascular disease

Hypertension during pregnancy is assessed relative to the individual patient's norm, an increase of 15 mmHg diastolic pressure over the patient's pre-pregnant or early pregnancy level being taken as significant. A blood pressure over 140/90 is routinely regarded as abnormal, and a level above 110 mmHg diastolic is regarded as severe. Fluid retention may only be evidenced by increased weight gain.

None of the signs of pre-eclampsia is specific; the diagnosis is made by the presence of more than one component. Hypertension and hyperuricaemia (the upper limit of plasma urate is 0.2 mmol/l at 28 weeks' gestation, rising to 0.39 mmol/l at 36 weeks) are early signs; proteinuria, coagulopathy, and liver and placental dysfunction occur late.

In some cases the mother presents primarily with liver damage, thrombocytopenia, and microangiopathic haemolysis, without the conventional markers of pre-eclampsia—the HELLP (haemolysis, elevated liver enzymes, low platelet count) syndrome, which may be confused with a medical or surgical condition (for example cholecystitis), and carries a relatively poor prognosis. Hypovolaemia is also associated with a poorer outcome.

The speed of progression of the disease varies from case to case. The danger of eclampsia is heralded by the patient's complaints of right hypochondrial pain, oliguria, shortness of breath, confusion, visual disturbances, or headache in the great majority of cases. Examination may show brisk tendon reflexes and clonus, retinal oedema, and retinal artery spasm. There may be focal neurological signs, the signs of pulmonary oedema, hepatic or uterine tenderness, or bleeding per vaginam. Eclamptic fits, which are of the grand mal type, may be preceded by tremor or facial twitching. Death is usually due to cerebral haemorrhage.

Laboratory tests should include full blood count (platelet count often low), uric acid, liver and renal function, clotting studies, blood grouping, and urinalysis. Chest X-ray and ECG are advisable. The fetus should be monitored. All pregnant women with a blood pressure above 140/90 should be referred to the duty obstetrician for consideration of admission. Extreme pre-eclampsia may need the commencement of treatment in the emergency department. The mother should be placed in a quiet, dim, calm environment, and oxygen should be given.

Hydralazine is the first-line treatment of severe pre-eclampsia. It may be given in intravenous boluses of 10 mg each 20 minutes, titrated against the fall in blood pressure, or as intramuscular boluses of 10 mg repeated each 2–3 hours combined with 500–1000 mg of methyldopa orally. Labetalol and diazoxide have been recommended as second-line drugs, and, more recently, nifedepine has been used safely and effectively. The aim is a diastolic pressure of 90–100 mmHg, to maintain the placental flow.

Intravenous fluid should be based on urine output plus c. 1500 ml/24hrs (more if in labour, or if vasodilators are administered). Patients who are hypovolaemic will need an initial fluid bolus.

Eclamptic fitting must be promptly controlled by intravenous diazepam 10 mg boluses repeated up to 5 times (fetal depression accompanies higher doses) or chlormethiazole 0.8 per cent solution given as an initial load of 40–100 ml, then infused at 60 ml/hr (fetal depression accompanies dosage over 1500 ml). Phenytoin 18 mg/kg should be given intravenously at a rate of 50 mg/minute to prevent further fits. The mother's electrocardiogram must be monitored during phenytoin administration. Rarely, paralysis and IPPV may be needed. Magnesium sulphate infusion is a routine first-line treatment in the United States; the aim is a plasma level of 4–7 mEq/l. Complications of its use include refractory hypotension, cardiac arrest, tetany, and neonatal respiratory depression.

When pre-eclampsia is severe, or eclampsia has supervened, the fetus should be delivered as soon as possible; even very premature babies stand a better chance of survival out than in. The mother will need urgent transfer to an obstetric unit with neonatal intensive-care facilities.

Disseminated intravascular coagulopathy complicates the picture in 7 per cent of cases.

Hepatic rupture presents with the onset of shock, in a patient with right hypochondrial pain and raised LFTs. As it is fatal in 70 per cent of cases, laparotomy is imperative.

Uterine rupture may present ante-partum, where the cause is separation of a uterine scar from a previous operation, but is now exceedingly rare, having been more common when classical Caesarean section, with a vertical incision in the upper uterine segment, was popular. The symptoms and signs may be subtle, the patient complaining of gradually increasing abdominal pain until the rupture becomes complete, in which case there is severe pain and shock. Laparotomy is imperative.

Further reading

Abell, T. L. and Riely, C. A. (1992). Hyperemesis gravidarum. *Gastroenterology Clinics of North America*, **21** (4), 835–49.

Brandjes, D. P., Schenk, B. E., Buller, H. R., and ten Cate, J. W. (1991). Management of disseminated intravascular coagulation in obstetrics. *European Journal of Obstetrics, Gynaecology and Reproductive Biology*, **42** (Suppl.), S87–9.

Demers, C. and Ginsberg, J. S. (1992). Deep venous thrombosis and pulmonary embolism in pregnancy. *Clinics in Chest Medicine*, **13** (4), 645–56.

Fraser, R. B. (ed.) (1990). Workshop on eclampsia. *Care of the Critically Ill*, **Vol. 6** (1), 6–23.

Redman, C. and Walker, I. (1992). *Pre-eclampsia: the hidden threat to pregnancy*. Oxford University Press.

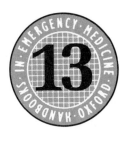

CHAPTER 13

The patient with a complication of labour or delivery

Key points in the patient with a complication of labour or delivery

1 The symptoms and signs of early pre-term labour are subtle. Increased uterine contractions, constant backache, pelvic pressure, increased urinary frequency, increased vaginal discharge which is bloody or watery, and diarrhoea have been found to be significant. Once congenital abnormalities are excluded, 85 per cent of all perinatal fatalities are subsequent to pre-term labour.

2 The clinical diagnosis of premature rupture of the membranes (PROM) is difficult and tests for amniotic fluid must be performed as soon as the diagnosis is suspected. The essence of management of PROM is to minimize the risk of ascending infection and give the fetus its maximal chance to mature *in utero* if the PROM is significantly pre-term. Vaginal examination should therefore be performed using a sterile speculum. Digital examination should be avoided as it may induce labour as well as introduce infection.

3 The prolapsed cord should be routinely sought after the rupture of membranes, where associated factors mean the risk of prolapse is high, or there is evidence of fetal distress. Perinatal mortality is 20–30 per cent. Effective, immediate action is imperative if the baby is to survive.

4 Fetal distress presents with meconium staining of the liquor and/or fetal heart rate abnormalities. One tenth of deliveries reveal meconium stained liquor; fresh green staining is the warning sign. Management should be directed at relieving the cause where possible or expeditiously delivering the baby, often by Caesarean section.

5 In the first stage of a breech presentation labour, cord prolapse should be sought and the passage of the head must be delayed until the cervix is fully dilated. Once the second stage is in progress, the principles of management are gentle handling of the fetus to avoid traction and compression injuries and controlled delivery of the head.

6 The first baby of a twin delivery is delivered in the normal fashion except that the routine syntometrine injection accompanying delivery of the anterior shoulder must not be given. The delivery of the second twin must be effected in less than fifteen minutes. The delivery of the first twin is often followed by up to half an hour of uterine stand-still. Oxytocin infusion should accompany labour, with the dose being increased as necessary after the birth of the first child once the membranes surrounding the second twin have been ruptured.

7 Shoulder dystocia is defined as delivery of the head but impaction of the shoulders behind the symphysis pubis. This is a major obstetric emergency: 50 per cent of babies sustain asphyxia or birth trauma. Help must be summoned as soon as the diagnosis is suspected.

8 85 per cent of women who suffer an amniotic fluid embol-ism die. During delivery, or immediately post-partum, the mother becomes acutely short of breath, hypotensed, and may be cyanosed, fitting, or comatose. Intermittent posi-tive pressure ventilation, dopamine infusion, the reversal of metabolic abnormalities, and the treatment of coagulo-pathy must be rapidly instituted as required. The baby must be delivered immediately.

9 The signs of uterine rupture may be gross or subtle. Sus-picion should be raised by: persistent lower uterine pain and tenderness between contractions. There is usually bleeding p.v., and the fetus may be distressed. Uterine scar separation may be made manifest only by fetal dis-tress. The mother must be energetically resuscitated, then laparotomy performed to stop the bleeding.

10 Primary Post-partum Haemorrhage is defined as the loss of 500 mls or more of blood from the genital tract or placenta in the first 24 hours post-partum. When PPH has occurred, an intravenous infusion must be started, blood cross-matched and clotting studies sent, the duty obstetri-cian summoned urgently if they are not already present, and the duty anaesthetist alerted. The genital tract should be rapidly assessed for lacerations. If the uterus is atonic, it must be contracted by the use of fundal massage, and by

bolus intravenous Syntocinon, oxytocin 5–10 units, or ergometrine 0.25 mg, repeated, if necessary, twice more at twenty minute intervals.

11 Placental separation is indicated by apparent lengthening of the umbilical cord and by change in the uterine shape to a higher, rounder outline. If the placenta is separated but mechanically retained these signs should be present. Where the placenta is partially or completely adherent or unseparated these signs will be absent. Either situation may be accompanied by any degree of haemorrhage.

12 Complete uterine inversion presents with sudden and profound shock accompanied by a variable degree of external blood loss. The patient is in a variable degree of pain and may feel the need to 'bear down'. An attempt to revert the uterus should be made immediately the condition is recognized, without delaying for anaesthesia or removing the placenta.

13 Post-partum pelvic infection, which follows 5–10 per cent of deliveries, is often polymicrobial and is treated with a combination of antibiotics. Disseminated intravascular coagulation may supervene.

Pre-term labour

Pre-term labour is defined as labour commencing before 37 weeks of gestation. It affects 8 per cent of deliveries, of which 4–6 per cent are induced. Once congenital abnormalities are excluded, 85 per cent of all perinatal fatalities are subsequent to pre-term labour.

Bacteria may initiate labour by the production of a phospholipase which acts on the arachidonic acid of the amnion, increasing intrauterine prostaglandins; these then stimulate the uterus to contract. Abnormal bacterial colonization of the vagina, chorioamnionitis, and neonatal infection have been found to be associated with premature birth, but there is as yet no unequivocal evidence for the efficacy of antibiotics in prolonging the pregnancy.

The aetiology is summarized in Box 13.1.

Box 13.1 **Aetiology of pre-term labour (spontaneous onset only)**

- previous pre-term delivery
- second-trimester abortion
- smoking
- low socioeconomic class
- multiple pregnancy
- polyhydramnios
- uterine anomaly
- cervical incompetence
- pyelonephritis
- genital-tract infection
- abruptio placentæ
- trauma
- high maternal fever

The symptoms and signs of early pre-term labour are subtle. Increased uterine contractions, constant backache, pelvic pressure, increased urinary frequency, increased vaginal discharge which is bloody or watery, and diarrhoea have been found to be significant. The patient may, however, be unaware of contractions, and when contractions are noticed they are often neither frequent nor painful.

In later gestation, in nearly all cases the baby is 'better out than in'. The decision may be made to use a beta-sympathomimetic infusion to allow time for the transfer of the patient to a more suitable facility or the administration of steroids to encourage fetal lung maturation. Ritodrine may be used, and is infused at 0.05 mg/minute initially and augmented by 0.05 mg/minute until the contractions cease or the dose reaches 0.35 mg/minute. The infusion is then maintained at the minimum effective dose for 24 hours. A 500 ml bolus of Ringer's lactate should be infused first. Where the fetus's chance of survival is slim, ritodrine is commenced as above, but is continued as oral medication until 36 weeks' gestation. The side-effects of ritodrine include hypotension, tachycardia, hypokalaemia, hyperglycaemia, pulmonary oedema, and a raised serum lactate. The volume of fluid given should be carefully controlled and monitored. Ritodrine can be given as a 3 mg/ml solution in a syringe pump or an 0.3 mg/ml solution in a standard IV pump; 5 per cent dextrose should be used as the diluent.

Magnesium sulphate is a routinely used tocolytic in America. Indomethacin is also effective, but pulmonary hypertension and premature closure of the ductus arteriosus are associated with its use in late pregnancy. It is suggested that it should be used only where gestation is less than 32 weeks. Nifedepine is a recently suggested alternative to β-agonists which appears useful and well tolerated.

Vaginal delivery should be conducted with great care, particularly with regard to the fetal head, as sudden compression–decompression changes as the head passes through the perineum may cause intracranial damage. Entonox or an epidural should be used for pain-relief. Episiotomy should be performed.

Every effort must be made to avoid delivery during a transfer. The travel time and likely progress of the labour must be evaluated, and ritodrine infusion should be initiated unless specifically contraindicated.

Premature rupture of the membranes

Premature rupture of the membranes (PROM) is defined as rupture of the membranes earlier than 37 weeks' gestation. It affects 2–3 per cent of deliveries, and is associated with polyhydramnios, cervical incompetence, and multiple pregnancy. Genital-tract infection and placental vasculopathy have been implicated. Clinical diagnosis may be difficult, as patients may present with a rush of fluid or a slow leak.

The essence of management of PROM is to minimize the risk of ascending infection and give the fetus its maximal chance to mature *in utero* if the PROM is significantly pre-term. Vaginal examination should therefore be performed using a sterile speculum. Digital examination should be avoided, as it may induce labour, as well as introducing infection. The examination must include exclusion of prolapse of the cord. Fluid may be seen passing through the cervical os. A yellow nitrazine stick dipped into the fluid will go black if liquor is present. Amniotic fluid will 'fern' on a laboratory slide. **It is vital that these tests are done as soon as the patient is assessed.** At the same examination, a vaginal swab should be taken for bacterial culture. The diagnosis of early infection is difficult: raised white counts, ESR, and C-reactive protein may help. Later infection is made manifest by pyrexia, purulent discharge, and uterine tenderness.

The patient should be admitted to a facility with a neonatal intensive-care unit for rest and observation, with induction of labour if signs of infection occur, if there is oligohydramnios, or at 34–37 weeks.

If labour starts spontaneously beta-sympathomimetics should only be tried to cover transfer of the mother to a suitable unit for delivery.

PROM may be complicated by cord prolapse, all the consequences of prematurity for the infant, and intrauterine infection of the fetus. Where oligohydramnios has developed delayed delivery may result in limb deformities. Pulmonary hypoplasia affects up to 20 per cent of infants; its prevalence seems related to the gestational age of the fetus at the time of PROM.

Cord prolapse

'**Cord prolapse**' arises when part of the umbilical cord lies below the fetal presenting part. It affects 0.25–0.5 per cent of deliveries. Perinatal mortality is 20–30 per cent. Fetal asphyxia may leave the baby neurologically impaired. The aetiology is summarized in Box 13.2.

Box 13.2 Aetiology of cord prolapse

- Premature rupture of membranes
- Premature fetus
- Malpresentations
- Fetal deformity
- Multiple pregnancy
- Polyhydramnios
- Placenta praevia
- Pelvic malformation and tumours
- Iatrogenic (for example during version)

The prolapsed cord should be routinely sought after the rupture of membranes, where the factors in Box 13.2 apply or where there is evidence of fetal distress. **Effective, immediate action is imperative if the baby is to survive.**

Cold or careless manipulation of the cord can cause vasospasm. First, therefore, the cord is gently cradled in the palm of the hand and replaced in the vagina. The tips of the fingers of the cradling hand are used to push the presenting part away from the cervix. The effect of gravity must be neutralized by tipping the bed head-down and elevating the mother's buttocks above her chest either by kneeling or the combination of pillows with the lateral position. The traditional approach is to maintain this combination of attendant's hand and maternal position until the baby can be delivered (this may include transfer to a suitable facility) by Caesarean section, or forceps-assisted vaginal delivery if the cervix is fully dilated and the presentation is cephalic. Recently, some practitioners advocate replacement of the cord into the uterus followed by vaginal delivery (funic replacement). If the baby is already definitely dead or non-viable, normal labour and delivery may be allowed; but the benefit of the doubt must always lie in the child's favour.

Fetal distress

Fetal distress presents with meconium-staining of the liquor and/or fetal heart-rate abnormalities. One-tenth of deliveries reveal meconium-stained liquor; fresh green staining is the warning sign. The fetal heart usually beats between 120 and 160 times per minute, with periodic changes in response to uterine contractions and fetal movement. The absence of this normal variability combined with a persistent fetal tachycardia is indicative of hypoxia.

Deceleration occurring other than in the early part of the contraction (which is due to a fetal vagal response to compression of the head) may be ominous. Slowing of the fetal heartbeat to less than 120 bpm should be carefully evaluated— a fall to less than 100 bpm may indicate a need for urgent intervention. Deceleration patterns may defy classification; but three types have been characterized as indicative of fetal distress. 'Late' decelerations start at the peak of the contraction and persist after its end. They are usually attributable to a decrease in the supply of oxygen to the placenta associated with excessive uterine action or maternal hypotension. 'Prolonged' decelerations persist for two minutes or more. 'Variable' decelerations vary in timing and length, those lasting longer than sixty seconds having prognostic implications. They are thought to be due to cord compression. The persistence of a 'variable' pattern for more than fifteen minutes may indicate hypoxia. The combination of baseline loss of variability and tachycardia with these ominous patterns of deceleration increases the likelihood of hypoxia. In cases of doubt fetal scalp blood samples may be tested for acidosis. The aetiology is outlined in Box 13.3.

Management should be directed at relieving the cause where possible or expeditiously delivering the baby, often by Caesarean section. Syntocinon should be stopped, any

---

Box 13.3 **Aetiology of fetal distress**

- Decreased placental flow due to:
    - Excessive uterine contraction (syntocinin, abruption)
- Hypotension (APH, epidural, IVC compression, drugs):
    - Vasoconstriction (hypertension)
    - Idiopathic placental 'dysfunction' (small-for-dates fetus)
- Decreased umbilical cord blood flow due to:
    - Cord compression
    - Cord prolapse
- Maternal hypoxia due to:
    - Eclampsia
    - Epilepsy
    - Anaemia
    - Cardiac disease
    - Respiratory disease
- Fetal anaemia (for example Rhesus isoimmunization)
- Fetal exsanguination due to:
    - Vasa praevia
    - Preferential flow to another fetus in multiple pregnancies

---

hypotension corrected, vaginal examination performed, and oxygen, reassurance, and pain-relief administered to the mother. Turning the mother on her side will relieve compression of the inferior vena cava. Raising the buttocks may relieve cord compression. Intravenous terbutaline (0.25 mg) bolus may be used to abolish uterine contractions in acute intra-partum fetal distress in selected patients.

Breech presentation

Abnormal presentations are largely diagnosed antenatally, when appropriate plans for delivery are made. When a patient presents in labour and the presentation is unusual, the obstetrician must be contacted immediately. However, the emergency physician should have a rudimentary knowledge of the method of delivery where the fetus has passed into the birth canal, as events may outstrip the speed of the obstetric team.

Breech presentations are defined as *frank* when the fetal buttocks present and the legs are extended, as *flexed* when the buttocks present and the legs are flexed, and as *footling* when the foot presents: 4 per cent of deliveries are breech, with prematurity being a particular risk factor.

In the first stage, cord prolapse should be sought, and a careful assessment of the cervix must be made, as the breech may pass through before full dilatation is reached. The passage of the head must be delayed until this has happened. This may be effected by epidural anaesthesia and lifting the breech cranially *per vaginam*.

Once the second stage is in progress the principles of management are gentle handling of the fetus, to avoid traction and compression injuries, and controlled delivery of the head. Asphyxia results from cord compression, or from delay in delivery. Intracranial damage is caused by compression–decompression forces resulting from uncontrolled delivery of the head. Cervical spine and brachial plexus injuries can result from heavy-handed traction or hyperextension of the neck during delivery. Limb fractures and dislocations can follow entrapment and inappropriate manœuvres. Damage to internal organs can attend manipulations.

The three sections of the delivery are the spontaneous descent of the buttocks; the rapid, gently-assisted delivery of the trunk; and the forceps-controlled slow delivery of the head. The detail of the delivery of the fetus depends on the position of legs and arms.

An episiotomy should be performed once the perineum is *distended* by the breech; flexed legs may be hooked down easily once the buttocks are spontaneously delivered; extended legs can be released by flexing first the anterior, and then the posterior, leg at the knee. The abdomen will follow; any tension on the accompanying cord must be released.

Once the head reaches the pelvic brim the fetus becomes hypoxic; delivery is therefore imperative within three minutes. The back is kept anterior, the attendant's hands are used to cradle the fetal pelvis, and the uterine contractions are allowed to expel the trunk to scapula level. Flexed arms are pulled down by passing two fingers over each shoulder to sweep the arms down across the chest. If the delivery of the baby stops after the thorax, the arms may be extended. Extended arms may be delivered by rotating the thorax so that one shoulder is beneath the mother's symphysis pubis and then sweeping the first arm across the front of the thorax. The thorax is then rotated through 180° and the other arm delivered in a like manner. At this stage the fetus is allowed to dangle until the occipital hairline is in view. The baby's body is then lifted carefully to the horizontal, freeing the face and allowing the baby to breathe. The head is then best delivered under forceps control. The baby's body is lifted upwards and the blades applied beneath it, the blade to the left side of the mother being applied first, then the right. Traction should be gently applied.

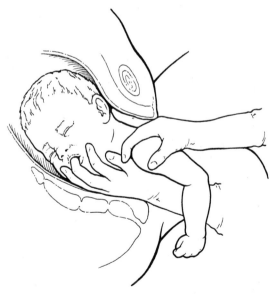

Fig. 13.1 • Delivery of the after-coming head.

If delay in the second stage occurs, retraction of the vagina applied to the baby's face (for instance with a forceps blade) will allow the baby to breathe.

If the head arrests at the pelvic brim, the fetus should be held as shown in Fig. 13.1. The mouth finger flexes the head, and gentle traction is applied with the index and middle fingers of the other hand on the shoulders, rotating the head if necessary so that the back of the baby's neck lies under the pubic arch, until the chin is delivered. The face is then carefully guided slowly over the perineum. During the delivery of a breech any rotation of the back posteriorly must be reversed. After delivery, the mother must be carefully checked for trauma of the genital tract. Cervical lacerations are particularly common, owing to the tendency of the breech to descend before the cervix is fully dilated.

Multiple pregnancy

Multiple pregnancies are relatively rare in Caucasians, but more common in Afro-caribbeans, older women, those of high parity, and those who have taken drug therapy to aid conception. Twins occur in 1:90 deliveries, triplets in 1:10 000 and quadruplets in 1:500 000: 45 per cent present as vertex/vertex, 35 per cent as vertex/breech, 10 per cent as breech/breech, and 10 per cent as tranverse/vertex or transverse/breech. As many as 5 per cent of twin pregnancies are missed on booking ultrasound scans. The emergency physician may therefore be faced with a precipitate expected or unexpected multiple delivery.

Pre-term labour, cord prolapse, and post-partum haemorrhage may result. The delivery of the first twin may be accompanied by shut-down or partial separation of the placental bed, or followed by exsanguination of the second twin by preferential blood flow to the first where there are anastamotic placental connections. The perinatal mortality is 15 per cent. The overdistended uterus may contract poorly. The delivery of the first twin is often followed by up to half an hour of uterine standstill.

Episiotomy is routinely performed, and the first twin is

delivered in the normal fashion **except that the routine syntometrine injection accompanying delivery of the anterior shoulder must not be given.**

The delivery of the second twin must be effected in less than fifteen minutes. The second fetus should be continuously monitored. Oxytocin infusion should accompany labour, with the dose being increased as necessary after the birth of the first child once the membranes surrounding the second twin have been ruptured.

Any transverse lie should be externally turned to vertex or breech before the membranes are ruptured. If there are complications such as cord prolapse or fetal distress the birth will need to be assisted by forceps or section. If the lie is transverse and external version was unsuccessful, the child may be turned by grasping the feet through the membranes and pulling it round into a breech.

If syntometrine was given with the anterior shoulder, the twin pregnancy having been missed, the second twin must be delivered within three minutes by the use of forceps, breech extraction, and internal version as indicated.

The delivery of the last baby should be followed by 5 units of oxytocin intravenously and continued oxytocin infusion.

Shoulder dystocia

Shoulder dystocia is defined as delivery of the head but impaction of the shoulders behind the symphysis pubis. It occurs in 0.25 per cent of deliveries. The cause is mechanical mismatch between fetus and mother's pelvis. Large babies, those who are post-mature, and those who are born to mothers with a small pelvis or diabetes are at risk.

Instead of entering the pelvis obliquely, the fetus attempts to pass through the antero-posterior diameter and impacts between pubic symphysis and sacrum. The fetus asphyxiates due to chest and cord compression.

This is a major obstetric emergency: 50 per cent of babies sustain asphyxia or birth trauma. Help must be summoned as soon as the diagnosis is suspected. Suggestive features are slow crowning of the baby's head, and difficult in delivering the face by extension. Spontaneous rotation of the head does not occur, and normal traction does not deliver the anterior shoulder.

A large episiotomy must be made. If the anterior shoulder has passed the pelvic brim, a firm pull in the normal direction whilst the mother hyperflexes her hips and an assistant pushes suprapubically may shift the shoulder. If this does not work in fifteen seconds, a hand should be inserted between neck and symphysis and the fetus rotated by pressure on the anterior surface of the posterior shoulder so that the shoulders lie obliquely. If these techniques fail, a hand is inserted intravaginally along the chest and the posterior fetal forearm and hand are grasped. The arm is delivered by sweeping it across the chest anteriorly. If the fetus is still impacted, rotate the anterior shoulder to posterior and, if necessary, repeat the arm-delivery manœuvre.

Post-partum haemorrhage and genital tract trauma are associated. A careful check of the mother must be made after the third stage.

Amniotic fluid embolism

Amniotic fluid embolism occurs during or just after about 1:5000 deliveries: 85 per cent of mothers who suffer an amniotic fluid embolus die.

The aetiology is summarized in Box 13.4.

Box 13.4 Aetiology of amniotic fluid embolism

- Multiparity
- Strong uterine activity
- Operative delivery
- Polyhydramnios
- Abruptio placentæ

Acute pulmonary vascular obstruction causes acute pulmonary hypertension, which stresses the heart, causing a fall

in cardiac output. There is a pulmonary ventilation–
perfusion imbalance. During delivery, or immediately post-
partum, the mother becomes acutely short of breath, and
may be cyanosed, fitting, or comatose. Vaginal bleeding becomes torrential as disseminated intravascular coagulation
supervenes. There is hypotension and may be pulmonary
oedema. Chest X-ray shows no specific change, and lung
scans exhibit diffuse patterning. Intermittent positive-
pressure ventilation, dopamine infusion, the reversal of
metabolic abnormalities, and the treatment of coagulopathy
must be rapidly instituted as required. The baby must be
delivered immediately. Cardiopulmonary resuscitation may
be necessary.

Uterine rupture

Uterine rupture accompanies 1:3000 labours. It may be complete or incomplete, leaving the visceral peritoneum intact.
The aetiology is summarized in Box 13.5. The prognosis is
worse when the rupture occurs in an intact uterus than when
it is due to separation of a uterine scar.

Box 13.5 **Aetiology of uterine rupture**

- obstructed labour (especially in the multiparous)
- uterine operative scar
- oxytocin/prostaglandin E2
- obstetric manœuvres (for instance internal version; forceps)
- trauma (for example during road-traffic accidents)
- termination of pregnancy
- multiparity
- placenta accreta/percreta
- cornual pregnancy
- concealed abruptio
- uterine anomaly
- trophoblastic disease

The signs of rupture may be gross or subtle. Suspicion should be raised by persistent lower uterine pain and tenderness between contractions. There is usually bleeding *per vaginam*, and the fetus may be distressed. Uterine scar separation may be made manifest only by fetal distress. Swelling and crepitus may be found over the lower uterus, and haematuria may be noted. The mother may be hypotensed and tachycardic.

Box 13.6 **Aetiology of post-partum haemorrhage**

- Failure of uterus to contract/retract: 80–90 per cent of PPH
  ——for atonic reasons:
    —Multiple pregnancy
    —High parity
    —Big baby
    —Placenta praevia
    —Polyhydramnios
    —Lengthy third stage
    —Precipitate labour
    —Deep anaesthesia
    —Full bladder
  ——for mechanical reasons:
    —Retained placenta
    —Retained clots
    —Fibroids
    —Uterine anomalies
- Genital-tract trauma
  —Episiotomy
  —Lacerations: cervix, vagina, perineum
  —Uterine rupture
  —Caesarean section
- Pregnancy-induced hypertension
- Coagulopathy
- Uterine inversion
- Amnionitis

Complete rupture presents with severe pain and shock, fetal death, recession of the presenting part, and bleeding *per vaginam.*

The diagnosis is confirmed by manual exploration of the uterus.

The mother must be energetically resuscitated; then laparotomy should be performed to stop the bleeding, and the surgeon should proceed to hysterectomy or repair as indicated. If transfer to a more suitable unit is desirable and the patient can be stabilized, she must be transferred with intravenous lines in place, and accompanied by trained staff and cross-matched blood. The application of a MAST suit may buy time.

Primary post-partum haemorrhage

Primary post-partum haemorrhage is defined as the loss of 500 ml or more of blood from the genital tract or placenta in the first 24 hours post-partum. It follows 2–6 per cent of deliveries (20–25 per cent recurrent). The aetiology is summarized in Box 13.6.

Prophylaxis is provided for routine births by intramuscular injection of syntometrine with the delivery of the anterior shoulder. Oxytocin 5 units IM should be used in preference if the mother has heart disease or hypertension. Where there is a high risk of PPH, oxytocin or ergometrine may be given intravenously with delivery of the anterior shoulder; or an infusion of oxytocin (10–20 units/500 ml) may be started.

When **PPH has occurred**, an intravenous infusion must be started, blood must be cross-matched and samples for clotting studies sent, the duty obstetrician must be summoned urgently if not already present, and the duty anaesthetist must be alerted. Where there is considerable haemorrhage, central venous pressure and urine output monitoring will be needed. The genital tract should be rapidly assessed for lacerations, and a bimanual assessment should be made of the tone of the uterus. If it is atonic, the uterus must be contracted by the use of fundal massage, and by bolus intravenous oxytocin 5–10 units, or ergometrine 0.25 mg, repeated if necessary at twenty-minute intervals twice more. Fundal massage is performed by gently rubbing the uterus with a hand placed on the patient's abdomen, putting the thumb in front of, and the fingers behind, the fundus. Retained clots should be firmly massaged out.

If the uterus remains atonic, an oxytocin infusion of 20 units in 500 ml crystalloid may be run as fast as is necessary to retain uterine contraction up to a maximum of 100 milliunits/minute. Retained products must be manually removed under spinal or general anesthesia.

If the haemorrhage continues despite these measures, carboprost (15-methyl PGF2α) 0.25 mg may be given intramuscularly, and repeated at intervals between 15 minutes and 90 minutes (depending on the extremity of the patient's condition) up to a total dose of 12 mg. Intravaginal PGE2 may also be effective.

If bleeding persists and operative intervention is not rapidly available, bimanual compression of the uterus may be performed. One fist is placed in the anterior fornix, pushing the uterus upwards. The second hand is placed abdominally behind the fundus and pulls the uterus forward, compressing it against the vaginal hand. This may be combined with rotatory massage. Uterine packing may be a useful holding measure.

In refractory cases hysterectomy or hypogastric or uterine artery ligation or embolization may be indicated to control the bleeding. Embolization or vasopressin infusion of the bleeding pelvic vessels identified by angiography may be a possible conservative alternative.

Sheehan's syndrome is infarction of the anterior pituitary gland in association with PPH where significant hypovolaemia has been allowed to occur. The presence or absence of lactation in the postpuerperium must be carefully monitored.

Specific conditions giving rise to PPH include retained placenta, genital-tract trauma, and uterine inversion.

Retained placenta

Delay in the delivery of the placenta can be defined as a third stage which exceeds thirty minutes. The placenta is usually delivered 5 to 10 minutes after the baby. **Retained placenta** affects 2 per cent of deliveries. Where the placenta has separated from the uterine wall, its retention is due either to uterine atony or to a constriction ring. The placenta is adherent to the uterine wall in placenta accreta, increta, and percreta, although non-pathological adherence also occurs. The placenta separates from the uterine wall as its bed becomes too small for it as the uterus contracts. This process is accompanied by retroplacental bleeding. Haemostasis after delivery of the placenta is effected by the smooth muscle lattice of the uterus contracting to compress the torn vessel endings. A defective ability of the uterus to contract or a mechanical block to such contraction will allow continued bleeding after full placental separation. The three grades of placental adherence are defined as follows: *accreta*: the placenta adheres to the myometrium; *increta*: the placenta invades the myometrium; and *percreta*: the placenta penetrates to the serosal layer.

Placental separation is indicated by apparent lengthening of the umbilical cord and by change in the uterine shape to a higher, rounder outline. If the placenta is separated but mechanically retained these signs may be accompanied by a degree of bleeding from mild to torrential. Where the placenta is partially or completely adherent or unseparated these signs may be absent. Again the degree of bleeding varies from case to case.

The separated placenta is withdrawn by the Brandt–Andrews method. If the uterus is atonic the general measures outlined above are applied. A contraction ring can be felt as a tight band; fluothane or cyclopropane anaesthesia should relax it sufficiently for withdrawal of the placenta.

Where the placenta has not separated, and haemorrhage is slight, treatment may initially be expectant. Where the the patient already has epidural blockade removal may be effected after 10 minutes. In other cases, if the placenta has not separated in 30 minutes, removal under GA or epidural is indicated. Where facilities for this do not exist the patient should be transported with an oxytocin infusion *in situ* (20 units in 500 ml crystalloid) to the nearest appropriate unit. If at any time the bleeding becomes heavy removal should be effected. The placenta will need to be removed manually whenever there is significant haemorrhage unresponsive to oxytocin. The procedure should be performed under general anaesthesia or epidural blockade. Where the extremity of the patient's condition and the available facilities make it unavoidable then local anaesthetic blockade and inhalation anaesthesia may be used.

To remove the placenta manually, one hand is used to put light tension on the cord while the other traces the cord up to the placenta. The first hand is then placed on the abdominal wall, pushing down the fundus, whilst the inner hand is held in a spade shape (fingers and thumb aligned and together) and used to blunt dissect the placenta from the uterine wall through the decidua spongiosa. Once it is completely separated, **and not before**, the placenta is grasped firmly and carefully withdrawn from the uterus. A speedy manual exploration of the uterine wall for retained fragments of placenta or uterine wall damage should follow. If pieces of placenta have been left behind there are considerable risks of haemorrhage and infection.

Placenta accreta can usually be manually stripped; there will be no palpable plane of cleavage in increta, and hysterectomy is unavoidable where there is haemorrhage.

The lower genital tract should then be checked for trauma and treated accordingly.

Genital-tract trauma

Most **lower genital-tract bleeding** is due to lacerations of the perineum, vagina, or cervix. Haematomata are more common following instrumentation or precipitate labour. They may be vulval, paravaginal, in the broad ligament, or retroperitoneal. Haematomata of the broad ligament are associated with rupture of the lower uterine segment.

Lacerations should always be sought once the third stage is complete. Bleeding from lacerations of the lower vagina, vulva, and perineum should be controlled by direct pressure until repair can be effected. Continued oozing from vaginal or cervical lacerations may require packing, followed by repair under general anaesthetic.

Brisk haemorrhage from a cervical tear may be controlled by clamping the cranial end of the tear with sponge forceps. Such tears should be properly explored and sutured in theatre.

Haematomata of the vulval area give rise to severe pain, and are evident clinically, usually shortly after delivery. They may be more significant than suspected as a result of extension into the paravaginal and/or ischiorectal spaces. Those of the paravaginal area present with pain, retention, tenesmus, and restlessness. Examination *per vaginam* reveals a tense swelling. Haematomata of the broad ligament may be felt on bimanual palpation, and may displace the uterus laterally. Retroperitoneal haematomata may rupture into the peritoneal cavity, causing life-threatening hypovolaemia. Intravenous fluids should be started and blood should be cross-matched. Any surgical intervention will require general anaesthetic. Vulvar and paravaginal haematomata are incised and evacuated, and bleeding points are stabilized. Catheterization and vaginal packing may be required for 24 hours. Broad ligament haematomata may be treated conservatively unless bleeding appears to be continuing, when laparotomy, rarely accompanied by hysterectomy or internal iliac ligation, will be required.

Uterine inversion

Uterine inversion is defined as incomplete if the uterine fundus is inverted but does not herniate through the cervix, and complete if the fundus herniates through the cervix, lying in the vagina or externally. It follows 0.02 per cent of deliveries. Fundal insertion of the placenta is a predisposing factor. The shock which accompanies complete inversion has both neurogenic and hypovolaemic components. The neurogenic element is caused by traction on the intra-abdominal structures.

The aetiology is summarized in Box 13.8.

Box 13.8 Aetiology of uterine inversion

- Third-stage mismanagement—fundal pressure or cord traction performed before uterine retraction
- Traction on an adherent placenta
- Abrupt increase in intra-abdominal pressure before uterine retraction (for example from vomiting)
- Short umbilical cord, or cord wrapped around the baby
- Inappropriately fast withdrawal of the placenta during manual removal

---

Incomplete inversion may present with a palpable notch in the top of the uterus felt abdominally, or may become evident on exploration for the cause of post-partum haemorrhage. Rarely, it may be missed until it progresses to complete inversion. Complete inversion presents with sudden and profound shock, accompanied by a variable degree of external blood loss. The patient is in a variable degree of pain, and may feel the need to 'bear down'. Intravenous fluids should be instituted and blood cross-matched. An attempt to revert the uterus should be **made immediately the condition is recognized**, without delaying for anaesthesia or removing the placenta. Delay will allow the formation of the cervical ring and swelling of the uterus. Oxytocic agents must be withheld until the uterus is reverted. The fundus is cupped in the hand and pushed cerebrally, with countertraction by ring forceps on the cervix if needed.

The position is held for three minutes. If still present, the placenta is then removed manually and cautiously withdrawn. Ergometrine 500 micrograms is given, an oxytocin infusion is instituted, and the patient is carefully checked over the next few hours. If this first attempt fails, the next attempt should be made under general anaesthesia, within one hour of the inversion. Manual and hydrostatic methods may be tried. Where these are unsuccessful surgical correction will be needed.

Uterine inversion is a dire condition. The maternal death rate is high where facilities are limited. The third stage must, therefore, be meticulously managed, and attempted reversion must never be delayed.

Other post-partum problems (secondary haemorrhage, psychological symptoms, psychosis, and infections)

Secondary post-partum haemorrhage is defined as fresh bleeding 24 hours to six weeks post-delivery. It follows 1 per cent of deliveries. The aetiology is summarized in Box 13.9.

Box 13.9 Aetiology of secondary post-partum haemorrhage

- Retained placental fragments
- Intra-uterine infection
- Genital-tract trauma
- Fibroid
- Chronic uterine inversion
- Trophoblastic disease

The main management decision in these patients lies with the obstetrician, and is whether to explore the uterus. Patients presenting with a minor bleed may settle or may progress to torrential haemorrhage. Augmentin may be started to cover sepsis. Patients with frank haemorrhage, poor health, or poor social circumstances should be admitted. Heavy bleeding should be urgently referred to the duty obstetrician; an intravenous infusion should be instituted and syntocinon (0.5–1.0 ml IV) should be given.

Sepsis, subinvolution, or the degree of bleeding may necessitate early exploration. Ultrasound may help distinguish between other cases. Exploration must be performed cautiously, with intravenous lines in place, as severe haemorrhage may accompany the procedure. Operative complications include haemorrhage necessitating hysterectomy for control, and uterine perforation.

Post-partum, psychological symptoms are the norm; enervation, irritability, tearfulness, and anxiety being common around the fourth day (the 'baby blues'). Up to 10 per cent of women need formal treatment for postnatal depression, those who have previous affective illness being particularly at risk.

Post-partum psychosis follows 1:1000 deliveries, being more common in those who have suffered a previous episode. The incidence and severity of the condition are often underestimated by assessing physicians; the association with suicide, infanticide, child abuse, and marital breakdown make it a major post-partum emergency. Patients present three to four days post-partum with an acutely psychotic picture of confusion, delusions, hallucinations, or mania. Organic causes should be excluded, and acute psychiatric referral should be arranged.

Post-partum pyrexia is defined as day-long pyrexia of more than 38 degrees on any two of the days two to ten post-partum. A rise in temperature during labour, or at the onset of lactation on day three, may be regarded as normal. The pyrexia may be due to urinary-tract infection, chest infection, local wound infection, mastitis, thrombophlebitis, coincident systemic illness, or pelvic infection. A full examination, including fauces, legs, perineum, and breasts should be made. Urine specimens and vaginal and cervical swabs should be taken. Blood culture should be performed where there is a possibility of septicaemia.

Post-partum infection should always be assumed to be pelvic in origin until proved otherwise. Those who have undergone a long labour, endured a sizeable passage of time from rupture of the membranes to birth, or had multiple vaginal examinations during labour, and those who are poorly nourished are at greater risk.

Post-partum pelvic infection follows 5–10 per cent of deliveries. It is fatal in 5 per cent of cases. Infections are often polymicrobial; common causative organisms include *Streptococcus, Staphylococcus, Clostridium perfringens, E. coli, Klebsiella, Proteus,* and *Bacteroides faecalis.* Associated factors are summarized in Box 13.10.

Box 13.10 Factors associated with post-partum pelvic infection

- Caesarean section
- the passage of time since rupture of the membranes
- trauma from for example internal version, forceps, or episiotomy
- possibly internal monitoring, or repeated examinations *per vaginam*
- socio-economic classes IV and V

The initial endomyometritis may spread to the nearby reproductive structures or to the pelvic peritoneum, and may cause pelvic cellulitis, intraperitoneal abscesses, pelvic thrombophlebitis, or frank peritonitis. More virulent organisms can cause septicaemia. Rarely, septic emboli from a streptococcal infection may cause lung abscesses. *Clostridium perfringens* may present with jaundice due to haemolysis, and may rapidly prove fatal. Disseminated intravascular coagulation may complicate the infection.

The patient presents with pyrexia, backache, abdominal pain, and uterine tenderness, which may be accompanied in more severe cases by foul lochia, subinvolution, and the signs of local spread or peritonitis. The perineum, vagina, and cervix must be carefully inspected for lacerations. An abscess is evidenced by variable pyrexia, vomiting, ileus, pain, and a tender pelvic mass. Persisting pyrexia and a perivaginal mass are characteristic of pelvic cellulitis. Septicaemia may be unaccompanied by local signs. Subinvolution and significant bleeding should raise the possibility of retained products of conception.

Local swabs and blood are taken for culture. A baseline haemoglobin level should be taken, and if bleeding is continuing or the level is low, blood transfusion may be needed.

An infusion of oxytocin may be started where bleeding is significant. Treatment should be commenced forthwith as outlined in Box 13.11. Breast-feeding may be contraindicated by the antibiotics used.

Box 13.11 **Treatment of suspected post-partum pelvic infection**

Vaginal delivery:
Mild symptoms—ampicillin or co-trimoxazole.
Severe cases—intravenous ampicillin, gentamicin, metronidazole.

Caesarean delivery:
Intravenous ampicillin and gentamycin routinely; add metronidazole if severe.

Septic shock:
As above for severe cases; also removal of the septic focus. Infusion/transfusion guided by CVP ± left atrial pressure monitoring. Dopamine may be used. Metabolic abnormalities need correction. Respiratory support may be needed, and DIC may supervene.

Abscesses:
Require operative drainage

Necrotizing fasciitis:
As for septic shock. Debridement of the whole of the involved area is indicated.

Mastitis is usually seen in those who are breast-feeding; cracked nipples are the route of infection. Stasis due to incomplete emptying and poor hygiene are contributing factors.

Staphylococcus causes most infections; *Streptococcus* and *E. coli* may be found.

The patient presents with fever, and local 'tumor, dolor, rubor, and calor'. The milk should be cultured, the breasts fully emptied, and flucloxacillin instituted. Breast-feeding should continue. Abscesses should be incised and drained under general anaesthesia.

Sutures in an **infected episiotomy** should be removed if there are any collections of pus. Augmentin should be prescribed when there is surrounding cellulitis. Salt baths and the use of a heat lamp are advised.

Marked cellulitis or lymphangitis should be referred to the obstetrician.

Further reading

Al-Azzawi, F. (1990). *A colour atlas of childbirth and obstetric techniques.* Wolfe Publishing, London.

Barrett, J. M. (1991). Funic reduction for the management of umbilical cord prolapse. *American Journal of Obstetrics and Gynaecology,* **165**(3), 654–7.

Brown, C. L., Ludwiczak, M. H., Blanco, J. D., and Hirsch, C. E. (1993). Cervical dilatation: accuracy of visual and digital examinations. *Obstetrics and Gynaecology,* **81**(2), 215–16.

Copper, R. L., Goldenberg, R. L., Davis, R. O., Cutter, G. R., Dubard, M. B., Corliss, D. K. *et al.* (1990). Warning symptoms, uterine contractions, and cervical examination findings in women at risk of pre-term delivery. *American Journal of Obstetrics and Gynaecology,* **162**(3), 748–54.

Management of post-partum haemorrhage (1992). *Drugs and Therapeutics Bulletin,* **30**(23), 89–92.

Iams, J. D., Stilson, R., Johnson, F. F., Williams, R. A., and Rice, R. (1990). Symptoms that precede pre-term labour and pre-term premature rupture of the membranes. *American Journal of Obstetrics and Gynecology,* **162**(2), 486–90.

Katz, M., Goodyear, K., and Creasy, R. K. (1990). Early signs and symptoms of pre-term labour. *American Journal of Obstetrics and Gynecology,* **162**(5), 1150–3.

Lewis, D. F., Major, C. A., Towers, C. V., Asrat, T., Harding, T. A., and Garite, T. J. (1992). Effects of digital vaginal examination on latency period in pre-term premature rupture of membranes. *Obstetrics and Gynaecology,* **80**(4), 630–4.

Maclean, A. B. (1990). Puerperal pyrexia. In *Clinical infection in obstetrics and gynaecology* (ed. A. B. Maclean), pp. 195–209. Blackwell Scientific Publications, Oxford.

Masson, R. G. (1992). Amniotic fluid embolism. *Clinics in Chest Medicine*, **13**(4), 657–65.

Morales, W. J., Smith, S. G., Angel, J. L., O'Brien, W. F., and Knuppel, R. A. (1989). Efficacy and safety of indomethacin versus ritodrine in the management of pre-term labour: a randomised study. *Obstetrics and Gynaecology*, **74**(4), 567–72.

Murray, L. (1992). Puerperal mental disorder. In *Obstetrics in the 1990s—current controversies* (ed. T. Chard and M. P. Richards), pp. 220–31. Blackwell Scientific Publications, Oxford.

Parer, J. T. and Livingston, E. G. (1990). What is fetal distress? *American Journal of Obstetrics and Gynecology*, **162**(6), 1421–5 (discussion, 1425–7).

Phelan, J. P. (1990). Uterine rupture. *Clinical Obstetrics and Gynaecology*, **33**(3), 432–7.

Rosemond, R. L., Lombardi, S. J., and Boehm. F. H. (1990). Ferning of amniotic fluid contaminated with blood. *Obstetrics and Gynaecology*, **75**(3, Part 1), 338–40.

Shekarloo, A., Mendez-Bauer, C., Cook, V., and Freese, U. (1989). Terbutaline (i.v. bolus) for the treatment of acute intrapartum fetal distress. *American Journal of Obstetrics and Gynecology*, **160**(3), 615–18.

Symposium on the third stage of labour and postpartum haemorrhage (ed. H. Gordon), (1990). *Journal of Obstetrics and Gynaecology*, **Vol. 10** (Suppl. 2).

Van Geijn, H. P., Copray, F. J., Donkers, D. K., and Bos, M. H. (1991). Diagnosis and management of intrapartum fetal distress. *European Journal of Obstetrics, Gynaecology, and Reproductive Biology*, **42** (Suppl.), S63–72.

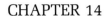

CHAPTER 14

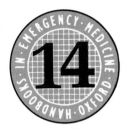

Obstetric procedures

Key points in obstetric procedures

1 In normal vaginal delivery, maternal and fetal trauma are minimized by slow, careful delivery of the fetal head.

2 Towards the end of the first stage, and in the second stage, entonox should be offered about half a minute before the next contraction is expected, to allow time for the gas tension in the central nervous system to build up enough to give analgesia.

3 Pethidine takes up to an hour to work if given intramuscularly. It is preferable to give intravenous aliquots of 20–25 mg at five-minute intervals until pain-relief is adequate.

4 A gush of blood from the introitus is an indication that the vaginal wall is tearing, and episiotomy is required.

5 Forceps delivery should be performed only if the correct conditions for their use pertain, and must be applied with great attention to technique.

6 The pre-requisites for post-mortem delivery are a viable fetus and a mother in whom resuscitation after sudden death is not possible or has failed; no attempt should be made when the mother has asphyxiated. Speed is of the essence, and delivery should ideally be complete within ten minutes of the mother's arrest.

Normal delivery

Labour and delivery is divided into three stages; the first stage from the onset of true labour until the cervix is fully dilated, the second from full dilatation until the baby is born, and the third from birth until the placenta and membranes are delivered and the uterus has retracted. The routine management of the first stage of labour is outside the remit of the emergency physician.

The descent of the head during the second stage of labour first distends the perineum with each contraction, and then leads to opening of the anus. The caput becomes visible, but recedes between contractions. Once the caput no longer recedes, the head has passed the pelvic floor and the baby is about to be born. The delivery of the head must be carefully controlled to maintain flexion of the head whilst it emerges and to prevent a sudden expulsion. One hand is laid on the top of the head and used to control the speed of emergence, whilst the finger and thumb of the other are laid either side of the anus, pressing gently through the perineum to maintain the flexed position until the biparietal diameter has passed, when the face may be delivered by carefully controlled extension. Maternal trauma is minimized by slow careful delivery of the head, and, once the head is crowning, the mother should be told not to push but to take rapid shallow breaths.

Immediately the head is born, the physician should feel around the neck with a finger to ensure that the cord has not become looped around it. If the cord is around the neck, it may be slipped forward over the head. If this is not possible, it must be clamped and cut at this stage.

The shoulders then rotate round into the antero-posterior diameter of the pelvis, and the next contraction should deliver first the anterior, and then the posterior shoulder. Such delivery must again be carefully controlled to avoid maternal trauma, and may be performed between contractions with the mother assisting with a series of voluntary small pushes. If the shoulders do not rotate after the birth of the head, gentle digital pressure may rotate them. If the anterior shoulder does not present, the neck of the baby may be bent gently towards the anus to bring it under the pubic arch. The posterior shoulder may then be delivered by bending the neck towards the mother's head. If these manœuvres still do not deliver the shoulders, a finger may be hooked into the axilla of the anterior shoulder to pull the shoulder down gently, or the posterior arm may be brought down by flexing it at the shoulder and elbow. All such manœuvres must be performed gently and with great care to avoid damage to the brachial plexus. Syntocinon 5 units, ergometrine 500 micrograms or syntometrine 1 ampoule (i.e. 500 micrograms ergometrine plus 5 units syntocinon) should be given as the anterior shoulder is delivered, to reduce post-partum haemorrhage.

Once the shoulders have been delivered, the trunk and legs follow rapidly. The baby should be kept at or below the level of the placenta until it has cried and pulsation in the cord has ceased, when the cord may be clamped with two artery forceps fifteen cm from the baby's umbilicus and cut between the clamps.

Separation of the placenta is indicated by 'lengthening' of the umbilical cord, rising up and contraction of the uterus, and a gush of blood *per vaginam*. It may be palpated in the vagina. The placenta is then removed by the 'Brandt–Andrews' method. The right hand holds the umbilical cord taut with artery forceps while the left hand, placed on the abdominal wall just above the pubic symphysis lifts the uterus cranially. The left hand then pushes downwards gently on the placenta until it is expelled, the right hand maintaining the cord taut. If the membranes do not follow the placenta, they may be gently pulled away with artery forceps.

The placenta and membranes should be inspected to ensure that they are complete, and the mother's perineum examined for trauma.

Anti-D Ig must be given if the mother is not Rh D immune and the child is Rh D positive, or if the mother will leave before the child's status will be known.

Analgesia for labour and delivery

The choice of **analgesia for labour and delivery** includes inhalation anaesthesia, local or regional anaesthesia, narcotics, and general anaesthesia. Other non-pharmacological methods may also be effective in the first stage: these include relaxation and breathing techniques, hot baths, and transcutaneous nerve-stimulation devices.

The emergency physician's involvement in labour is most likely to be limited to the late first stage and the second and third stages.

Nitrous oxide/oxygen gas mixtures can give effective analgesia at this stage of delivery when used correctly. The guiding principle is to allow for the time taken for the gas tension in the central nervous system to build up enough to give analgesia. In the first stage the patient should start breathing as the contraction becomes palpable, not when the contraction begins to hurt. Towards the end of the first stage, and in the second stage, this may not allow enough time, and the entonox should be offered about half a minute before the next contraction is expected. The gas is best self-administered, leaving the mother in control of her labour and ensuring safety, as she will drop the mask if she becomes drowsy.

Narcotic agents provide good pain-relief for many women. However, if the usual regime of administering 50–100 mg of pethidine intramuscularly is adopted, it should be remembered that it takes up to an hour for the drug to reach its most effective level. Giving 20–25 mg aliquots intravenously at five-minute intervals until there is adequate pain-relief is preferable. The effect is maximal within five minutes, and lower doses of narcotic are generally used, carrying less risk to the fetus. If the injection is given just as a contraction starts, this further diminishes drug delivery to the fetus, as placental flow is at its lowest. Ideally narcotics should be avoided altogether within two hours of delivery; however, should they be needed, naloxone should be given to the mother in the second stage.

Local anaesthetic infiltration of the perineum and vagina is sufficient to cover the procedure of episiotomy and the repair of simple perineal and vaginal lacerations: 10–15 ml of lignocaine 1 per cent are used. The dose administered must not exceed 5 mg/kg. Early signs of toxicity include tingling around the mouth, numbness of the tongue, dry mouth, muscle twitching, agitation, wooziness, and tinnitus. Fitting and cardiorespiratory depression may ensue. The convulsing patient should be placed on her side, the airway guarded, oxygen given, and the fits controlled with intravenous diazepam. Occasionally, paralysis and ventilation are needed.

The above methods will be insufficient to control pain if forceps delivery is planned. Pudendal nerve blockade is a safe, relatively simple method which, combined with the use of Entonox, gives reasonable pain-relief. A 20 cm 20 gauge needle is used. The ischial spine is felt through the vaginal wall using two fingers; these are then used to guide the tip of the needle through the vaginal wall and sacrospinous ligament so that it lies just below, and medioposterior to, the ischial spine. The plunger is withdrawn to confirm that the needle is not lying within a blood vessel; then 5 ml of lignocaine are injected. The needle is advanced 1 cm and another 5 ml are injected after checking for intravasation. The procedure is repeated on the other side. Local anaesthetic infiltration of the vulva (beginning at the fourchette and injecting well forward into the labia majora) may be combined with the block. If the vaginal approach cannot be used owing to the position of the presenting part, the transperineal approach may be used. Again, the ischial spine is located transvaginally; the needle is inserted half-way between the anus and the ischial tuberosity, directed towards the ischial spine; and lignocaine injected as before.

Episiotomy

Episiotomy should be performed for the indications summarized in Box 14.1. A gush of blood from the introitus is an indication that the vaginal wall is tearing. Midline perineal tearing is an indication for urgent episiotomy to protect the anus.

If there is no pre-existing regional or general anaesthesia, 10 ml of 1 per cent lignocaine should be infiltrated in the intended line of incision. The incision is best made postero-laterally to avoid the anal sphincter, and should be performed at the height of a contraction. An absorbable suture should be used for repair, with a continuous suture intra-vaginally extending from the cranial end of the incision (which should be carefully sought) to the vulva. Interrupted sutures are then used for the perineal body and interrupted or subcuticular sutures repair the perineal skin.

Box 14.1 **Indications for episiotomy**

- Delay in the second stage when the head is pressing on the perineum
- Threatened extensive perineal tear
- Fetal distress when the fetus has reached the perineum
- Previous complete perineal tear/prolapse repair
- Preterm delivery
- Forceps delivery
- Breech presentation
- Late prolapse of the cord

Forceps delivery

Forceps delivery is used for delay in the second stage of labour (see Box 14.2), maternal or fetal distress, pre-term delivery, and delivery of the head in a breech presentation. Maternal distress includes emotional exhaustion; physical signs are dehydration, tachycardia, and mild pyrexia. The emergency physician should hopefully be able to reach an obstetrician for help in most of these situations, but may be faced with delay in the second stage, when the top of the baby's head is clearly visible and no obstetric help is immediately available. Most of such delays are due to resistance of the pelvic floor, and the performance of an episiotomy will allow delivery. However, the assistance of forceps will be needed in some cases. Forceps should not be used unless the conditions outlined in Box 14.3 pertain. Their use carries the risk of laceration, haemorrhage, and infection for the mother, and intracranial haemorrhage, cephalhaematoma, and facial palsy for the neonate. Absolute attention must be paid to the correct application of the forceps to the biparietal diameter in vertex presentations and the bitemporal diameter in mentoanterior presentations. If there is doubt about the presentation due to scalp swelling, an ear should be sought; the position of the pinna should then make the baby's lie clear. The sagittal suture must always occupy the midline. The obliquity of the head must not exceed 45°. Attempts at extraction must always be gentle, with slow, intermittent traction of no more than moderate force.

The mother is prepared by emptying the bladder (catheterization may be necessary), swabbing the perineum with antiseptic, and towelling the surrounding area. Wrigley's short curved forceps are suitable for low forceps deliveries. The blade to the left-hand side of the mother is applied first. The practitioner's right hand is passed beside the fetal head, and the blade is guided between it and the fetal head. Initially the handle of the blade is held in the left hand, well over the mother's abdomen and almost parallel to her right inguinal ligament. As it is inserted the handle moves downwards and leftwards, coming to lie in the midline. The blade to the mother's right is then applied similarly. The handles should now appose and lock. Any resistance to meeting or locking implies a malapplication or malpresentation: the forceps must be removed and the fetal position checked. The inappropriate application of force will result in fetal trauma and possibly death.

The baby is then extracted by intermittent traction in a backwards and downwards direction in the axis of the birth canal. As the head reaches the outlet the handles rise to about 45°; as the head crowns they should be vertical. Each pull should last for no more than a few seconds. Once the head has crowned, the forceps should be removed and the face delivered by manual extension of the head. The rest of the delivery follows as routine, particular care being paid to the post-partum inspection of the genital tract for trauma.

The use of forceps in breech delivery is described in Chapter 13.

Box 14.2 Causes of delay in the second stage

- Resistant perineal floor
- Large baby
- Inadequate uterine contractions and voluntary effort
- Occipito-posterior, face, or brow presentations
- Deep transverse arrest of the head
- Small pelvic outlet

Box 14.3 Conditions necessary for the use of forceps

- Presentation vertex, face or breech
- If the presentation is face, the chin must be anterior.
- If the presentation is breech, the forceps are only used to deliver the aftercoming head.
- Head engaged
- Cervix fully dilated
- Membranes ruptured
- Bladder empty
- Uterus contracting
- Pelvic outlet adequate

Post-mortem Caesarean section

The pre-requisites for post-mortem delivery are a viable fetus and a mother in whom resuscitation is not possible or has failed. Sudden death of the mother carries the best chance for the child; no attempt should be made where the mother has asphyxiated. The next-of-kin should be informed, and permission obtained where possible; but this must not delay the procedure.

Cardiac massage and ventilation should be continued whilst the delivery is effected. Speed is of the essence, and delivery should ideally be complete within ten minutes of the mother's arrest. The prognosis after twenty minutes is very grim. Preferably, an obstetrician should operate; but the emergency physician must be prepared to proceed rather than incur any delay.

An incision is made from pubis to epigastrium through to the peritoneal cavity. The uterus is incised vertically for two inches just above the bladder reflection; then the uterine wall is elevated away from the fetus with the separated fingers of one hand, and the incision extended between the fingers to the fundus; an anterior placenta should be incised. The fetus is then delivered, and held, head tipped down, below the level of the mother's abdomen; and the cord is promptly tied and cut. The neonate should be kept warm, resuscitated as necessary, and transferred to a neonatal unit.

Further reading

Al-Azzawi, F. (1990). *A colour atlas of childbirth and obstetric techniques*. Wolfe Publishing, London.

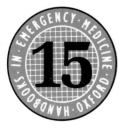

Care of the newborn infant

Key points in the care of the newborn infant

1 Routine suctioning of the oropharynx should be reserved for neonates where the airway is genuinely compromised by blood, liquor, or meconium, as overzealous suctioning may provoke apnoea.

2 The baby cannot maintain its own temperature at birth, which may drop by up to three degrees; a drop below 36 degrees should be avoided by the rapid provision of external warming.

3 The vast majority of babies who require resuscitation will respond to simple measures such as drying, warming, gentle stimulation, and 'blow-by' oxygen. Only a few will require advanced life-support procedures.

The normal newborn

During its time in utero the fetus makes 'breathing' movements which become more regular towards term. The fetal lungs contain about 30 ml/kg fetal weight of fluid. During birth this fluid is squeezed out of the airways, and the residue is absorbed across the alveolar walls. The change in fetal posture, the drop in ambient temperature, and the moderate hypoxia of birth all stimulate the baby's first breath. The maintenance of alveolar expansion is facilitated by the surfactant which is mainly produced after the thirty-second week of gestation. Where birth hypoxia is profound the central response to these stimuli may be depressed; breathing is then initiated by a primitive gasp reflex. Suctioning of the oropharynx, using a sterile manual mucus extractor with a user-protective modification, should be reserved for neonates where the airway is genuinely compromised by blood, liquor, or meconium, as overzealous suctioning may provoke apnoea.

In the fetus only 10 per cent of the cardiac output circulates through the lungs and pulmonary veins to the left atrium. Blood passing from the placenta in the umbilical vein is diverted from entering the portal vein by the ductus venosus and enters the inferior vena cava; as it enters the right atrium it largely streams through the foramen ovale into the systemic circulation. Blood flowing down the superior vena cava into the right atrium streams into the right ventricle and enters the pulmonary artery, where the large resistance afforded by the unexpanded fetal lungs causes it to be predominantly diverted to the aorta via the ductus arteriosus. The hypogastric arteries then form the last stage of the circulation back to the umbilical arteries and the placenta.

The expansion of the lungs by the first breaths causes the vascular resistance in the lungs to fall, and blood flow into the lungs is thus encouraged. It is thought that circulating fetal prostaglandins are broken down by the newly active lungs, and that these prostaglandins were necessary for the maintenance of the ductus arteriosus, which now contracts. The fall in pulmonary vascular resistance is paralleled by a rise in the systemic resistance as the placenta is replaced by the baby's peripheral circulation, which reverses flow across the foramen ovale. Over the next weeks the ductus arteriosus completes its closure by endarteritis, and the ductus venosus and umbilical vessels atrophy, the vein persisting as the ligamentum teres. The baby's cardiovascular system should be examined soon after birth, with particular reference to the heart sounds and femoral pulses. Weak femoral pulses may be indicative of coarctation of the aorta.

In utero the fetal temperature is dependent on that of its mother. Whilst the temperature regulatory centre becomes active immediately, the baby cannot maintain her own temperature at birth, which may drop by up to three degrees; a drop below 36°C should be avoided by the rapid provision of external warming. Labour should take place in a warm, draught free environment (ambient temperature at least 26°C), and once respiration has been established and the baby has been rapidly checked, she should be wrapped in warm towels. It is neither necessary nor wise to wash the newborn thoroughly at this time. The axillary temperature, which may vary normally from 36.0 to 37.2°C, should be periodically checked.

The initial assessment of the newborn baby is expressed as an Apgar score, which is computed by adding together scores allocated to five features of the newborn's state, ten being the maximal score. The scoring is outlined in Table 15.1.

Table 15.1 • Apgar score

Sign	0	1	2
Heart	absent	less than 100	more than 100
Respiratory effort	absent	slow, irregular	good, crying
Muscle tone	limp	some limb flexion	active
Response to stimulus	nil	grimace	vigorous cry
Colour	blue, pale	body pink, limbs blue	pink

A rapid external examination of the newborn baby should be performed, noting the presence of skin lesions, extra nipples or digits, sinuses or fistulae, abnormalities of the spine, mouth, palate, feet, genitalia, or anus. The head should be examined for scalp trauma, separation of the sutures, and areas of softening. Its circumference must be measured. The limbs should be checked for apparent fracture or paralysis. The abdomen may be rapidly felt. More detailed examination, including that for congenital dislocation of the hips and talipes, may be performed over the course of the next day or two, and is outside the remit of the emergency physician.

Resuscitation

A paediatrician should be routinely called to attend the deliveries listed in Box 15.1. Multiple births and the delivery of a baby of less than 31 weeks' gestation should be attended by two paediatricians, ideally accompanied by a nurse and a transport incubator from a neonatal intensive-care unit.

Box 15.1 **Call paediatrician for:**

- Forceps deliveries
- Meconium-stained liquor
- Fetal distress
- Breech deliveries
- Multiple births
- Pre-term deliveries
- Babies of diabetic mothers
- Post-mortem Caesarean sections
- Antenatally diagnosed congenital abnormalities

However, the child may be born before a paediatrician can attend, and the emergency physician should be prepared to resuscitate the newborn infant. Cord blood gases should be taken whenever the fetus has been distressed or is born prematurely. These are taken into heparinized syringes from both the umbilical vein and artery in a piece of umbilical cord which has been double-clamped eight inches apart.

The vast majority of babies who require resuscitation will respond to simple measures. Only a few will require advanced life-support procedures.

The baby must be born into a heated environment (ambient temperature 26°C or more), immediately dried, wrapped in warm towels, and placed under a radiant heater in a horizontal or slightly head-down position, with the neck extended about 10°. If the Apgar score is above 5 but breathing is absent or inadequate, the baby may be stimulated by gently flicking the soles of her feet, or rubbing her back gently with a towel. Blood, liquor, and secretions may be suctioned from the mouth and nose if necessary, taking care not to advance the suction catheter more than 5 cm past the lips. Oxygen at 2 l/minute is given from a mask held above the mouth and nose. High oxygen flow-rates should be avoided, as these may cool the baby.

If breathing remains inadequate into a second minute after birth, oxygen should be given by bag and mask, or by a mask connected to a resuscitaire with a Y-connector, at 30–40 breaths per minute. The operator should be careful to avoid compressing the baby's submental area with the fingers of the hand holding the mask, and the bag should be squeezed gently, with just sufficient pressure to ensure an adequate rise of the baby's chest. Babies weighing less than 1500 g (roughly 31 weeks' gestation) should be intubated at this stage, rather than maintained with a bag and mask. Oxygen should be administered through a system with adjustable pressure, and an automatic 'blow-off' at pressures above 30 cm H_2O. Pressures of up to 30 cm H_2O and an inspiratory duration of two seconds may be needed for the initial breaths. Once the lungs are expanded, full-term babies may be maintained on 10–15 cm H_2O. If adequate chest rise cannot be obtained with a bag and mask, or apnoea persists into the third minute, the baby should be intubated.

Naloxone may be helpful if the mother has had a narcotic analgesic within four hours of delivery (10 micrograms/kg intravenously, repeated if necessary after three minutes, or 200–400 micrograms intramuscularly). Naloxone should NOT be given to the infants of opiate-dependent mothers.

The pulse rate can be judged by palpating the umbilical,

brachial, or femoral arteries, or by auscultation. Bradycardia will generally respond to improved oxygenation; however, if the rate remains less than 60–80 beats per minute, or the pulses are difficult to feel, external cardiac massage should be commenced.

If the initial Apgar score is below 5, or the baby is born dead, but the fetal heart was heard in the ten minutes preceding birth, the infant must be immediately resuscitated with intubation, ventilation, and cardiac massage, at three compressions for each ventilation. The protocol for full resuscitation is summarized in Box 15.2.

Box 15.2 **Protocol for full resuscitation of the newborn**

- Intubate orally, selecting tube size by the size of the nostril (usually size 2.5–3.0 for pre-term, 3.5 for term).
- Ventilate at 30 breaths per minute.
- Commence cardiac massage, with the fingers of both hands behind the spine and the thumbs compressing the lower chest 1–2 cm below the nipple line, at three compressions per inflation.
- If no immediate response, give 0.5 ml of 1:10 000 adrenaline via the ET tube.
- Place an umbilical venous catheter.
- Give 0.1 ml/kg of 1:10 000 adrenaline intravenously (repeat each 5 minutes).
- Give a bolus of 2 mmol/kg of 8.4 per cent sodium bicarbonate diluted with the same volume of 10 per cent dextrose (i.e. 6–10 ml of 8.4 per cent bicarbonate at term). If output returns, transfer to neonatal intensive care unit. If no response, consult a senior paediatrician about withdrawing treatment after twenty minutes.

Failure to respond may be due to:
- Malposition of the ETT.
- If the ETT is correctly positioned, block the valve on the ambubag for a few breaths (ONLY), and observe chest movement (some neonates need high initial

---

inflation pressures and a longer inspiratory time).
- Maternal analgesia with pethidine: give 200 micrograms naloxone (do NOT give if mother is an opiate addict) intramuscularly or 10 micrograms/kg intravenously.
- Ascites, pleural effusions, pneumothorax should be drained.
- Severe anaemia: give O-negative blood.

Life-threatening conditions presenting in the immediate post-partum period

Many malfunctions of the major systems or congenital defects may become evident over the first hours or days of the infant's life. The paragraphs below relate only to those abnormalities which may present in the first hour or two after birth.

Recurrent apnoeic attacks may be due to immaturity of the respiratory centres, but may also indicate intracranial damage, hypoglycaemia, or infection. Ventilation may be needed if the apnoea does not respond to simple stimulation as outlined above. Theophylline may be administered to decrease the severity and frequency of attacks.

Cyanosis may persist after birth despite the onset of respiration. Peripheral cyanosis is of no significance. Generalized cyanosis may result from respiratory, cardiac, or intracranial pathology. Where there is a respiratory cause the cyanosis lessens when the baby cries; where there is a cardiac or intracranial cause the cyanosis is unchanged or deepens with crying.

The passage of meconium is noted during up to 15 per cent of labours. The primitive gasp reflex may have already led to **meconium aspiration** in utero in some cases of asphyxia; immediate suction of meconium from the upper airway at birth before breathing is established may prevent meconium plugging of the distal airways, often complicated by pneumothorax and infection, which otherwise results. Box

15.3 summarizes the manœuvres to minimize the risk of aspiration.

Box 15.3 Manœuvres to minimize the risk of aspiration

- Call paediatrician and prepare resuscitaire.
- If the presentation is cephalic, suction the oro- and nasopharynx before delivering the shoulders.
- If the baby does not cry vigorously, hold the thorax firmly with the thumbs either side of the sternum to prevent gasping.
- Clear the oropharynx with suction and intubate.
- Using a size 6 suction catheter, suck meconium from the ETT, WITHDRAWING THE CATHETER AS YOU SUCK.
- Reintubate and repeat the process (up to five times) until no meconium is obtained.
- Stop chest clamping.
- If the baby still does not breathe vigorously, intubate and ventilate until pink and breathing normally.

The absorption of the last of the amniotic fluid across the alveolar membranes may be delayed. The baby will have rapid, shallow respirations, a 'grunt', and cyanosis (the **'transient tachypnoea of the newborn'**). The chest X-ray shows fluid in the horizontal fissure and some hazy shadowing. Warmth and oxygen directed towards the face are usually all the therapy that is needed, although the possibility of infection with Group B *Streptococcus*, which can present in exactly this way, should be considered. If symptoms persist beyond a few hours, blood cultures should be taken and penicillin and gentamicin treatment should be started.

Diaphragmatic herniation or eventration present with cyanosis, unilateral poor air entry, a displaced apex beat, and a 'scaphoid' abdomen. Ventilation will be needed, and a large nasogastric tube should be passed to keep the bowel deflated. Surgery is delayed until the baby is stable—often up to several days.

Other problems of respiration, such as hyaline membrane disease and pneumonia, do not usually become evident until a few hours postnatally; they are therefore outside the remit of this chapter.

Haemorrhage may occur during delivery from trauma to the placenta or cord; or the fetus may lose blood into the circulation of a twin or the mother. Significant bleeding will occur if the umbilical cord tie becomes loose. Birth pallor, coupled with a low haemoglobin, should be treated with immediate transfusion.

Jaundice in the first day of life is almost certainly due to haemolysis. Haemolytic disease occurs in 0.67 per cent of pregnancies. It is caused by antibodies which are raised against fetal red cell antigens (commonly Rhesus, A, or B) by the mother, and cross the placenta to bind to the infant's red blood cells, leading to their destruction by the fetal reticulo-endothelial system. Most cases are due to Rhesus incompatibility. Fetal blood cells cross the placenta in insignificant amounts during normal pregnancy, but during labour, and after abortion, ectopic pregnancy, or instrumentation (for example amniocentesis, termination of pregnancy) amounts sufficient to cause maternal sensitization to the fetal red cell antigen commonly mix with the maternal circulation. Such circulating fetal cells may be identified by the relative resistance of their haemoglobin to acid denaturation (the Kleihauer–Betke test). If prophylaxis is not given, haemolytic disease will affect the next pregnancy. The worst-affected fetuses die *in utero*, usually in the last trimester. Live infants are jaundiced and anaemic, with hepatosplenomegaly. The jaundice deepens postnatally, as the mother is no longer conjugating the bilirubin. High levels of unconjugated bilirubin cause kernicterus, which may lead to the child's death or to physical and mental incapacity in survivors. Haemoglobin, bilirubin, and reticulocyte levels are taken; the Coombs test is usually positive. The affected baby is treated with phototherapy, and exchange blood transfusion is performed if the haemoglobin is below 10 g/dl or the serum bilirubin is more than 120 micromol/l within twelve hours of birth. 160 ml/kg ('2 volume' exchange) of blood is slowly removed through the umbilical vein, and the same amount of blood lacking the antigen to which the mother was sensitized is transfused.

It is imperative that emergency physicians bear this most serious disease in mind when managing gynaecological and obstetric emergencies, in order to prevent rhesus immunization. Guidance on the use of anti-D immunoglobulin is given in Chapter 8.

The main role of the emergency physician in relation to **intracranial pathology** in the newborn is to minimize birth trauma and hypoxia. Massive intracranial haemorrhage or widespread ischaemic damage result in stillbirth or early death. Lesser degrees may present with hypotonia, bradycardia, apnoea, pallor or cyanosis, fitting, restlessness, drowsiness, dyskinesias, or fever, sometimes accompanied by a bulging fontanelle. The infant should be kept in a warm, quiet, darkened environment and handled as little as possible. Vitamin K must be given and phenobarbitone (a bolus of 20 mg/kg followed by 5 mg/kg/24 hours) may be used to control fitting.

Scalp haematomata must be looked for, and consideration must be given to any transfusion needs if such a lesion is large.

Difficult deliveries may result in **trauma** to the viscera, bones, or nerves. Whilst the last two can await later specialist advice, the first is life-threatening, and urgent transfusion and operative repair are indicated.

Hypoglycaemia presents with lack of interest and refusal of food, jitteriness or fitting, a fall in temperature, apnoeic spells, or coma. Infants at risk are pre-term, small- or large-for-dates, born to diabetic mothers, or stressed, or have been subject to placental insufficiency. Those infants who are symptomatic and belong to groups with low glycogen stores should be treated with a milk feed or intravenous glucose (5 ml/kg of 20 per cent glucose) depending on the degree of cerebral irritation. Those belonging to the islet cell hyperplasia group (large-for-dates and children of diabetic mothers) are best treated by milk feeds, but may have profound and prolonged hypoglycaemia requiring intravenous support. An infusion is better than repeated boluses. All at-risk babies should have frequent feeds initially.

Small-for-dates or pre-term babies may be **hypocalcaemic**, presenting with the clinical picture of neuromuscular irritability, hypertonia, and vomiting. If fitting is continuing, calcium gluconate 2.5 per cent in 5 per cent glucose solution is injected slowly until the fits stop (but not in excess of 4 ml/kg).

Vomiting is a non-specific indicator of disease in the newborn; but coupled with abdominal distension, and especially if there is bile present, it may indicate an **obstructive lesion of the gastro-intestinal tract**, such as a meconium ileus, small bowel atresia, or Hirschsprung's disease. Such a suspicion demands immediate abdominal X-ray and surgical consultation. Oesophageal atresia and tracheo-oesophageal fistula present with drooling and difficulty taking the first feed. Aspiration of the feed or stomach contents occurs. Failure to pass a catheter down the oesophagus confirms the diagnosis, and establishes the need to refer the baby immediately to a specialist paediatric surgical unit.

Infection acquired in the early postnatal period is usually derived from ascending vaginal flora, such as Group B *Streptococci*, or from transplacental infection with organisms such as *Listeria*. Early treatment is essential, as these infections carry a significant mortality even with antimicrobial therapy.

Further reading

Working Party of the British Paediatric Association (BPA), College of Anaesthetists, Royal College of Midwives, Royal College of Obstetricians and Gynaecologists (1989). *Resuscitation of the Newborn* (parts 1 and 2), pamphlet with video obtainable from The Royal College of Obstetricians and Gynaecologists, London.

June 1993 *Neonatal Resuscitation*, Report of a BPA Working Party (A. R. Wilkinson, Chair), pp. 1–22, British Paediatric Association, London.

PART 4
Background information

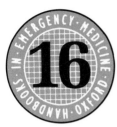

Anatomy and physiology

External genitalia (see Fig. 16.1)

The labia majora contain sebaceous, sweat, and apocrine glands. Their lateral aspects bear hair follicles. The round ligament terminates in the fatty core, which is continuous with the inguinal ligament. The canal of Nuck is formed by the persistence of an embryonic diverticulum of the peritoneal cavity which accompanies the round ligament into the inguinal canal. The labia minora contain sweat and sebaceous glands and erectile tissue. Bartholin's glands lie deep to the posterior ends of the labia minora and open into the vestibule. They secrete a mucus lubricant during sexual excitation, and may only be palpated if enlarged by tumour or inflammation. Similarly the duct orifices are only visible when inflamed.

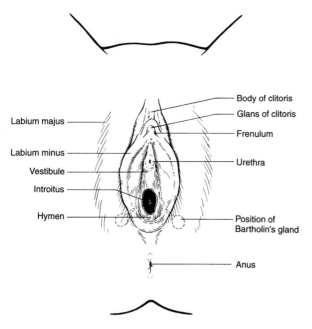

Fig. 16.1 • External genitalia.

Internal reproductive organs (see Fig. 16.2)

The vagina averages 10 cm in length. It is lined with squamous epithelium, which is rich in glycogen during the reproductive years, and produces a watery transudate. It is also lubricated by uterine and cervical gland secretions. Doderlein's bacilli produce lactic acid from the glycogen, causing an acid environment which restricts pathogens. The vaginal vault has posterior, anterior, and two lateral fornices, the deepest being the posterior, as the posterior vaginal wall is longer than the anterior.

The uterus is anteflexed in 80 per cent of women. The body of the adult uterus is 5 cm long; the cervix measures 2.5 cm and is lined by gland-containing columnar epithelium. The fundus is defined as that area of the uterus which lies above the openings of the fallopian tubes. The uterine wall consists of three layers of plain muscle; inner circular and outer longitudinal thin layers and a thicker middle layer full of blood vessels where the muscle

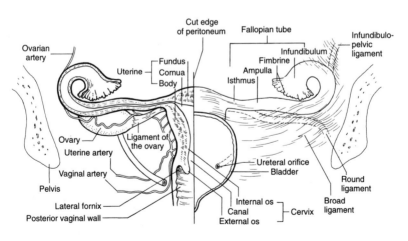

Fig. 16.2 • Internal reproductive organs.

bundles decussate. The vaginal surface of the cervix is lined with squamous epithelium, its central canal with columnar. The junction between these two cell types is usually at the external os, but may be advanced on to the vaginal surface. It is the site of origin of 95 per cent of cervical carcinomas.

The fallopian tube is 10 cm long and is divided into four parts: the interstitial portion lying within the uterine wall, the narrow isthmic area adjoining the uterus, the wide ampulla, and the terminal infundibulum. The infundibular opening is surrounded by frond-like fimbriae, one of which extends to partly embrace the ovary. The epithelium lining the tube consists of secretory and ciliated cells, and is pleated longitudinally.

The ovaries measure 3.5 cm in length and 2 cm in depth, and are 1 cm thick. Their position varies considerably. They are attached by their hila to the posterior surface of the broad ligament (a fold of peritoneum). Microscopically, the ovary consists of an outer layer of cubical cells lying on a layer of connective tissue, the tunica albuginea, surrounding the inner stroma of spindle-shaped connective tissue cells throughout which the Graafian follicles are scattered. During the reproductive years, some of the follicles mature, enlarge, and migrate to the surface of the ovary. In the middle of each menstrual cycle, one or more follicles rupture, releasing the ova and becoming corpora lutea. Each corpus luteum gradually regresses, becoming a hyaline corpus albicans. The structures of the follicle and corpus luteum are shown in Fig. 16.3. If conception occurs, the corpus luteum continues to grow until around the eighth week of gestation.

The ovarian ligament passes from the medial pole of the ovary to the uterus caudal to the fallopian tube. The round ligament runs from the same point on the uterus to the inguinal canal terminating in the labium majus. The pelvic fascia has two components. The parietal fascia lines the wall of the pelvic cavity and gives anchorage to the cardinal ligaments and levator ani. The visceral pelvic fascia forms the cardinal ligaments, which pass from the vaginal vault and cervix to the lateral pelvic wall, and are the main sup-

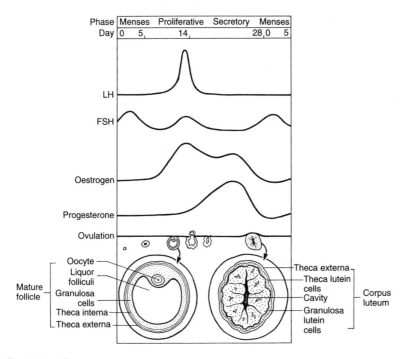

Fig. 16.3 • The menstrual cycle.

port for this area. The uterosacral ligaments are derived from the visceral fascia and run from the same area to the sacrum, giving support to the cervix. The bladder is also supported by condensations of the visceral fascia laterally and anteriorly.

Surrounding pelvic anatomy

The ovarian arteries arise directly from the aorta, inferior to the renal arteries. They run on the psoas major muscles to the pelvic brim, where they cross anterior to the ureters to enter the broad ligament. They supply the ovary and fallopian tube, and then anastomose with the uterine arteries.

The uterine artery arises from the internal iliac, running down the lateral pelvic wall and then turning medially in the base of the broad ligament to cross the ureter at the level of, and 2 cm lateral to, the internal os of the uterus. It gives branches to the cervix, upper vagina, and ureter, and then runs cranially beside the uterus, which it plentifully supplies, to anastomose with the ovarian artery.

The internal iliac artery also gives rise to the vaginal artery, the vesical arteries, which supply the bladder and ureter, and the pudendal artery, which supplies the perineum and vulva after leaving the pelvic cavity through the sciatic foramen. The rectum is supplied by superior, middle, and inferior haemorrhoidal arteries, arising from the inferior mesenteric, internal iliac, and pudendal arteries respectively.

The venous drainage comprises a series of plexi around the bladder, vagina, uterus, and rectum. The former three drain chiefly into the internal iliac veins, and the last into the inferior mesenteric veins as well as the internal iliac. The ovarian veins begin as double structures arising from a plexus within the broad ligament to run beside the ipsilateral ovarian artery. The double veins unite to form single vessels, the right of which drains into the inferior vena cava and the left into the left renal vein.

The lymphatic drainage of the internal reproductive organs passes to the iliac, obturator, and para-aortic nodes, whilst that from the vulva and perineum passes to the inguinal and superficial femoral nodes and then to deep femoral, iliac, obturator, and para-aortic nodes. The lymph then drains into the cisterna chyli at the level of the second lumbar vertebra to flow through the thoracic duct to the great veins at the base of the neck.

The sensory nerve supply of the perineum and vulva passes via the pudendal nerve to the second, third, and fourth sacral nerves, via the posterior femoral to the first, second, and third and via the ilioinguinal and genitofemoral nerves to the first lumbar root. The motor supply to the levator ani, anal sphincter, and superficial perineal muscles derives from the second, third, and fourth sacral nerves. The autonomic nerve supply of the internal organs is shown in

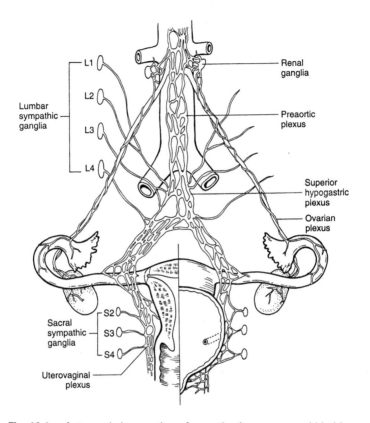

Fig. 16.4 • Autonomic innervation of reproductive organs and bladder.

Fig. 16.4. The function of the supply is uncertain. The awareness of pain arising from the pelvic viscera reflects this supply.

The muscles of the pelvic floor are shown in Fig. 16.5. The vagina is supported by the perineal and levator ani muscles and by the perineal body. The pubococcygeal portion of the levator ani maintains the angle between the posterior wall of the urethra and the bladder base. It relaxes to allow the bladder neck and upper urethra to descend and relax during micturition.

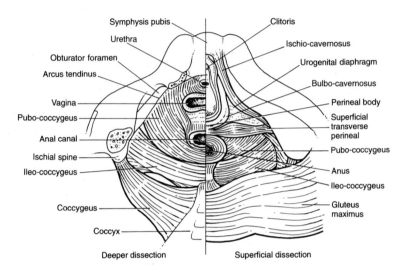

Fig. 16.5 • Muscles of the pelvic floor from below.

The menstrual cycle

Between one and two million primordial follicles are thought to be present in the ovaries at birth. Of these around fifty begin to mature with each menstrual cycle, but only one reaches full maturity. It does this under the influence of the hormone surges outlined in Fig. 16.3, p. 229. The hypothalamic gonadotrophin-releasing hormone (GnRH) is released in a pulsatile manner, leading to pulses of luteinizing hormone (LH) and follicle stimulating hormone (FSH). Oestrogen has varying effects on the pituitary response to GnRH, being inhibitory in the early part of the menstrual cycle and facilitatory in the middle part. Inhibin is produced by the follicles; it preferentially inhibits FSH secretion. The endometrial response to the hormone cycle is initially proliferative (follicular) and then secretory (luteal). During the follicular phase the stratum basale, the layer of endothelium lying next to the uterine muscle, is stimulated by oestrogen to grow cubical epithelium, which becomes replete with narrow, tubular glands and both straight and coiled arterioles. During the luteal phase the joint action of oestrogen and progesterone causes increasing convolution of the glands and arterioles. The inner layer of secretory epithelium is named the stratum compactum, that adjacent to the stratum basale, the stratum spongiosum. Both hormones' levels fall at the end of the cycle. The endometrium shrinks and is shed piecemeal, as it is stripped away by haemorrhage from necrosed vessel walls. This process is regulated by prostaglandins synthesized in the endometrium and myometrium under the influence of the premenstrual progesterone level fall. Prostaglandin F2α is a vasoconstrictor, prostaglandin E2 a vasodilator.

The menstrual cycle averages 28 days, but may vary normally between women from 21 to 35 days. Irregularities are common at menarche and menopause. Menstrual loss varies between individuals, and may normally contain small clots and endometrial debris. Significance is therefore to be found in any change of pattern. Premenstrual complaints include weight gain, headache, malaise, sore breasts, lower abdominal pain, and backache.

Puberty usually commences around the age of eleven with breast-bud enlargement, followed by pubic hair at the age of twelve and the menarche at thirteen. A range from 10 to 15 may be regarded as normal for the menarche.

The usual age of onset of the menopause lies between 47 and 52. The menstrual periods either stop abruptly, become lighter, or become less frequent. After the periods cease the uterus shrinks, the endometrium, vaginal wall, and vulva atrophy, the suspensory ligaments and fascia no longer adequately support the uterus, the labia flatten, and pubic hair growth diminishes. There is thought to be a hormonal basis for the flushing of the face and neck and sweating which are common at this time. Osteoporosis results from an increased urinary excretion of calcium attendant on the reduction in oestrogen levels, and there is a tendency to bone fractures.

The anatomy and physiology of pregnancy

The fimbrial end of the fallopian tube comes into contact with the ovary around the time of ovulation. The ovum enters the tube and is swept towards the uterus by the fluid produced by the ciliated cells, the action of the cilia, and peristalsis. Fertilization normally takes place in the ampulla. The ovum usually reaches the uterus about six days after ovulation.

The proliferative and secretory changes produced in the endometrium by the hormones of the normal menstrual cycle become more exaggerated after implantation of the ovum, and the endometrium is then named the decidua. When the ovum has implanted the decidua is divided into three parts: the decidua basalis between the ovum and the muscles of the uterine wall, the decidua capsularis between the ovum and the uterine cavity, and the decidua vera lining the rest of the uterus. The space between the latter two layers is called the decidual space, and that between the basalis and the chorionic villi the choriodecidual space. As the trophoblast invades the decidua, the endothelium of the maternal blood vessels is destroyed; then trophoblastic cells invade the walls, and the vessels are converted from narrow-ended structures into funnel-ended ones. The placental chorionic villi, therefore, are bathed in a lake of maternal blood which squirts in through about 200 arterioles and is collected into the decidual veins. The placenta is held to the uterus by anchoring villi where the trophoblast is in direct contact with the decidual plate.

The placenta is fully developed by the end of the first trimester; it continues to grow in depth up to 16 weeks' gestation, and in circumference in step with the fetus and uterus to term. At birth the average placenta weighs 500 g, and measures three cm in depth and 20 cm in breadth.

It is divided into about 20 cotyledons which are separated from each other by a shallow groove, each corresponding to a main villous stem containing a terminal branch of the umbilical artery. Each cotyledon is further divided into up to twenty lobules, each corresponding to the opening of a maternal vessel. The umbilical cord containing one vein and two arteries lying in Wharton's jelly is usually inserted at the centre of the placenta, but may be inserted at the edge (battledore placenta). The cord averages 50 cm in length.

The placenta is continuous with the chorion, both structures being lined on the fetal surface by amnion. The amnion is lined by cubical epithelium which secretes amniotic fluid in early pregnancy. As pregnancy progresses the volume of fluid is increased by diffusion through the fetal skin (up to twenty weeks) and membranes and, later, by fetal renal excretion. There is exchange across the membranes with maternal plasma, and some fluid is removed by fetal swallowing. By term the volume of fluid averages 800 ml; it contains sloughed fetal and amniotic epithelial cells. Both fluid and cells may be sampled via amniocentesis.

The uterine increase in size has three components: an increase in cell mass under the influence of oestrogen and progesterone; hypertrophy of the cells; and distension by the fetus and placenta. The wall has three layers: a thin inner concentric layer; a thick middle meshwork of fibres which constrict the interweaving blood vessels by contracting; and a thin outer layer which arches over the fundus. The glands of the cervix become distended with mucus; there is often an extension of columnar epithelium on to the surface of the cervix. Cervix, vagina, and vulva become significantly vascular. The blood supply to the uterus is markedly increased.

The mass effect exerted by the gravid uterus is summarized in Box 16.1. Ureteral dilatation is caused by the effect of progesterone as well as by compression by the uterus.

During pregnancy the corpus luteum is maintained by human chorionic gonadotrophin (HCG) produced by the trophoblast for 10 weeks or more, ensuring the production of oestrogen and progesterone to maintain the uterine decidua until the placenta is mature enough to take over. The corpus luteum then involutes. Oestrogen is secreted by the corpus luteum, the maternal adrenal glands, and the fetal adrenals and liver. The levels secreted rise throughout gestation, and are substantial. Hypertrophy and hypervascularity of the uterus, fallopian tubes, and vagina, proliferation of the

Box 16.1 **Mass effects of the gravid uterus**

The gravid uterus:
- displaces the diaphragm cranially by 4 cm;
- displaces the heart upwards and rotates it laterally;
- confines the small bowel to the upper abdomen;
- compresses the bladder, causing frequency in early and late pregnancy, impairing bladder emptying, and contributing to ureteral dilatation;
- causes 'supine hypotension' by decreasing venous return through compressing the inferior vena cava when the mother lies on her back; and
- contributes to the development of ankle oedema, varicosities of legs and vulva, and haemorrhoids by the same mechanism.

mammary duct system, and salt- and water-retention result. Progesterone is secreted by the corpus luteum and placenta. It causes preparation of the endometrium for implantation and proliferation of the alveolar tissue of the breasts if these structures have been previously primed by oestrogen. It is essential to the maintenance of pregnancy. HCG is abnormally high in multiple pregnancy and trophoblastic tumours. Prolactin is secreted by the anterior pituitary, and inhibited by dopamine from the hypothalamus, and initiates and maintains lactation in the ovarian-hormone-primed breast. Oxytocin from the posterior pituitary causes uterine contraction.

These hormonal changes are expressed in the symptoms and signs of pregnancy. Nausea is a common feature of the 6th to 14th weeks of pregnancy; appetite increases, a feeling of bloating is not rare, and heartburn is common. Gastric acidity is decreased, and there is a decrease in gastro-intestinal motility and gastric emptying. Constipation is often noted. The breasts enlarge, become knotty in texture, and tender, and the increased vascularity is evidenced by a network of veins under the skin. The nipples become prominent, the areolae dark, the sebaceous glands of the areolae enlarge (Montgomery's tubercles), and it becomes possible to express a clear fluid from the 12th week of pregnancy. Pigmentation of a line joining umbilicus and pubes is common (the linea nigra). The patient's forehead and cheeks may become pigmented, and spider naevi and palmar erythema may be seen. Stretch marks appear in two-thirds of pregnant women. The ligaments of the sacroiliac joints and symphysis pubis relax somewhat. The lower segment of the uterus feels softened on pelvic examination, and the cervix takes on a bluish tinge.

Physiological changes and laboratory data norms in pregnancy

The body adapts to pregnancy by the physiological changes summarized in Box 16.2 and 16.3.

Box 16.2 **Laboratory data norms in pregnancy**

- Haematocrit 32–41 per cent
- Haemoglobin 11–15 g/100 ml
- White cell count 5000–16 000/mm^3, but white cell counts as high as 25 000 may be a normal response to stress during labour and the puerperium.
- Platelets 134–400 thousands/mm^3
- Erythrocyte sedimentation rate 44–114 mm/hr
- Fibrinogen 4–6 g/100 ml
- Fibrin degradation products 14.0 ± 7.0
- pCO$_2$ 27–32 mmHg
- pO$_2$ 100–108 mmHg
- Bicarbonate 18–23 mmol/l
- Creatinine 38–90 micromol/l
- Urea 1.6–6.0 mmol/l
- Albumen 28–40 g/l
- Alkaline phosphatase rises through pregnancy: first trimester 33–87 iu/l, second trimester 31–117iu/l, third trimester 69–209 iu/l.

Box 16.3 **Physiological changes of pregnancy**

- Basal metabolic rate increases by up to 25 per cent.
- Blood volume increases by 30 per cent.
- Plasma volume reaches a maximal rise of around 50 per cent by 34 weeks.
- The red cell mass rises by 20 per cent.
- Pulse rate increases by up to 20 beats per minute.
- There is a decrease in peripheral resistance; diastolic blood pressure falls by as much as 15 mmHg during the first two trimesters, rising again to normal by term.
- Central venous pressure falls by 66 per cent by term.
- Cardiac output increases by up to 30 per cent (a systolic flow murmur may be heard).
- The electrocardiogram shows a left axis.
- Renal plasma flow and glomerular filtration rate increase steadily to an enhancement of 50 per cent by term.
- Pulmonary functional residual capacity falls, tidal volume increases, and minute ventilation increases by 40–50 per cent, oxygen requirements increasing by 20 per cent. (The 'hyperventilation of pregnancy'.)
- There is a slight depression in cell-mediated immunity, and auto-immune disease tends to remit in pregnancy.
- The anterior lobe of the pituitary hypertrophies.
- The secretion of both gluco- and mineralocorticoids is increased.
- The thyroid hypertrophies.

Further reading

Dewhurst, Sir J., de Swiet, M., and Chamberlain, G. (1992). *Basic science in obstetrics and gynaecology* (2nd edn). Churchill Livingstone, Edinburgh.

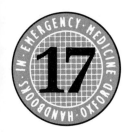

CHAPTER 17

Legal aspects

Consent to contraception

The National Health Service (Family Planning) Act of 1967 permitted local Health Authorities to provide family-planning services. Amendments to this Act mean that all methods of contraception, including sterilization, are legal in this country. The position of postcoital techniques remains controversial. At present the Law Officers' position is that there is no pregnancy until implantation is complete and that, therefore, postcoital methods which prevent implantation (the 'morning after' pill within three days and IUCD insertion within five days) are viewed as methods of contraception not abortion. Persons under the age of majority (18) may give consent to any medical treatment once they have reached the age of sixteen under the Family Law Reform Act 1969. A DHSS circular of 1980 advised practitioners that they could provide contraceptive treatment in exceptional circumstances to persons under sixteen without informing the parents. This was challenged through the courts, with the House of Lords eventually overturning a ruling by the Court of Appeal that such advice was unlawful. The Lords held that a person under sixteen may give a valid consent if of sufficient maturity and understanding. A doctor may, therefore prescribe contraception to girls aged less than sixteen if (i) s/he is satisfied that the girl can understand his/her advice; (ii) s/he cannot persuade the girl to inform her parents; (iii) the girl is likely to begin or continue sexual intercourse with or without contraceptive treatment; (iv) the girl's physical and/or mental health would suffer without contraceptive treatment; and (v) the girl's best interests require her/him to give contraceptive treatment and/or advice without the parents' consent.

Where the doctor thinks the girl is not sufficiently mature, there arises a conflict between confidentiality and the law. Each doctor must judge whether s/he feels it is in the best interests of the child to inform the parent against the child's wishes. The theoretical legal position that a doctor or parent providing, or consenting to, contraception for an under-sixteen could be regarding as aiding and abetting unlawful sexual intercourse has not been taken up by the judiciary.

Where a patient lacks the mental capacity to consent to contraception, there is no provision for another to consent for them under the Mental Health Act, as this only covers the treatment of mental disorder. The doctor may then act in the best interests of the patient as s/he sees them.

'Best interests' means that the doctor should act in a way which would be in accord with a responsible and competent body of relevant professional opinion.

No medical practitioner is *obliged* to prescribe any form of contraception against his/her beliefs.

Legal abortion (termination of pregnancy)

The governing legislation on abortion is the Abortion Act of 1967 as amended by the Human Fertilisation and Embryology Act 1990. Only the mother has the right to decide whether to seek an abortion; there is no paternal right under present legislation. The decision whether the sought abortion will occur is taken by two registered medical practitioners. Only a registered medical practitioner may terminate a pregnancy, although some of the procedures concerned (for example injection of prostaglandins) may be undertaken by another person under his/her direct authority. Abortions must be carried out in NHS hospitals or in premises approved for the purpose by the Minister. The amended Act allows abortion where the pregnancy has not exceeded its twenty-fourth week and it is the opinion of the two medical practitioners in 'good faith' that 'the continuance of the pregnancy would involve risk, greater than if the pregnancy were terminated, of injury to the physical or mental health of the pregnant woman. In determining ... such risk ... account may be taken of the pregnant woman's actual or reasonably fore-seeable environment.' Abortion is also allowed where the health of any existing children is put at risk, and where there is a substantial risk of the child's suffering serious handicap.

244 • Legal aspects

Pregnancy may be terminated when it is necessary to prevent grave permanent injury to the physical or mental health of the pregnant woman. Where such termination is 'immediately' necessary in the medical practitioner's opinion, the termination need not be agreed by a second practitioner or performed in an approved place. There is no legal gestational age-limit on the performance of abortions where there is a risk to the life of the mother, the risk of grave permanent injury to the mother, or the risk of serious handicap in the child. If an aborted fetus is born alive, the doctor is obliged to take reasonable measures to maintain that life, and may be prosecuted for failing to try to do so. No doctor is obliged to participate in any way in any abortion against his/her personal belief and conscience.

This legal position applies whether the abortion is surgical or is effected with mifepristone/gemeprost.

Still birth

The 'Still-Birth (Definition) Act 1992' came into effect on 1st October 1992. It reduced the minimum gestational age by which a still birth is defined from 28 weeks to 24 weeks. All babies born dead after 24 weeks' gestation, therefore, now require a still-birth certification. The parents of such babies can now pursue standard funeral arrangements, and Statutory Maternity Pay, Maternity Allowance, and Social Fund Maternity Payments may now be paid to qualifying mothers who gave birth to a stillborn child after 24 weeks' gestation.

Notification

1. To the Confidential Enquiries into Maternal Deaths

The Confidential Enquiries into Maternal Deaths require the notification of all deaths of women who were pregnant at, or recently before, their demise. Whatever the cause of death, therefore, all such deaths must be referred to the Coroner. In due course a form will be sent to the doctor who was in charge of the patient concerned requesting full and frank information regarding the death. The information collected is entirely anonymous and confidential.

2. Notifiable Diseases

Box 17.1 lists the presently statutorily notifiable diseases.

Box 17.1 **Statutorily notifiable diseases**

Cholera
Plague
Relapsing fever
Smallpox
Typhus
Acute encephalitis
Acute poliomyelitis
Anthrax
Diphtheria
Dysentery (Amoebic or Bacillary)
Leprosy
Leptospirosis
Malaria
Measles
Meningitis
Meningococcal septicaemia (without meningitis)
Mumps
Ophthalmia neonatorum
Paratyphoid fever
Rabies
Rubella
Scarlet fever
Tetanus
Tuberculosis
Typhoid fever
Viral haemorrhagic fever
Viral hepatitis
Whooping cough
Yellow fever

Further reading

Douglas, G. (1991). *Law, fertility and reproduction*. Sweet and Maxwell, London.

Appendix 1: Useful organizations

Assault

National bodies only are listed; each organization named has local units. Most police divisions now have Domestic Violence units, and some have (the rest should have access to) Rape Suites, the contact details for which should be obtainable from the local police station. Child Protection Team numbers, again, should be obtained from the local police station. The forensic medical examiner may be willing to collect evidence from victims of rape who do not at present wish to report the crime, for linkage with other cases, or in case the victim decides she wishes to prosecute at a later date; again the local police should know how to contact the FME.

Rape Crisis
PO Box 69
London
WC1X 9NJ
Help-Line: 071 837 1600

Victim Support (psychological and practical support for victims of crime)
National Office
Cranmer House
39 Brixton Rd
London SW9 6DZ
Tel.: 071 735 9166

Women's Aid (refuge, legal advice, and emotional support in cases of domestic violence)
Women's Aid Federation England
PO Box 391
Bristol BS99 7WS
National Helpline: Tel.: 0272 633542

Welsh Women's Aid
38–48 Crwys Rd
Cardiff CF2 4NN
Tel.: 0222 390874

N. Ireland Women's Aid
129 University St
Belfast BT7 1HP
Tel.: 0232 249041

Scottish Women's Aid
13 North Bank St
The Mound
Edinburgh EH1 2LP
Tel.: 031 225 8011

Child abuse

NSPCC
67 Saffron Hill
London
EC1N 8RS
National Help-Line: 0800 800500

Child-Line
National Help-Line: 0800 1111

Alcohol and drug abuse

(also refer to the drug and poisons information services listed in Appendix 2)

Alcoholics Anonymous: Welcome individual patients' calls.
National Help-Line: 071 352 3001

Alcohol Concern (source for information on local available help)
275 Gray's Inn Rd
WC1X 8QF
Tel.: 071 833 3471 (not for individual patient use)

Institute for the Study of Drug Dependence (offer information to professionals on any aspect of drug dependence and abuse, for example 'crack' in pregnancy; no personal counselling)
1 Hatton Place
London
EC1 8ND
Tel.: 071 430 1961/071 430 1993

Standing Conference on Drug Abuse (maintain list of all agencies dealing with drug abuse nationwide; offer information on local resources available)
1 Hatton Place
London
EC1 8ND
Tel.: 071 430 2341

Loss of fetus/child

Miscarriage
Miscarriage Association
PO Box 24
Offett
W. Yorks
WF5 9XG
Tel.: 0924 830515

Still birth
Still-Birth and Neonatal Death Society
28 Portland Place
London
W1N 5DE
National Help-line: 071 436 5881

Professional organizations

British Association for Accident and Emergency Medicine
The Royal College of Surgeons
35–43 Lincoln's Inn Fields
London WC2A 3PN
Tel.: 071 831 9405

The Royal College of Obstetricians and Gynaecologists
27 Sussex Place
London
NW1
Tel.: 071 262 5425

The Medical Protection Society
50 Hallam St
London
W1N 6DE
Tel.: 071 637 0541

The Medical Defence Union
3 Devonshire Place
London
W1N 2EA
Tel.: 071 486 6181

Appendix 2: Drugs and Pregnancy

Drugs/poisons information services: prescribing in pregnancy

The following information is reproduced from the 25th edition of the British National Formulary with the kind permission of the Pharmaceutical Press, Royal Pharmaceutical Society of Great Britain, and of the British Medical Association.

Drug Information Services

Information on any aspect of drug therapy can be obtained, free of charge, from Regional and District Drug Information Services. Details regarding the *local* services provided within your Region can be obtained by telephoning the following numbers:

England

Birmingham	021-311 1974	Direct Line
	or 021-378 2211	Extn 2296/2297
Bristol	0272 282867	Direct Line
Guildford	0483 504312	Direct Line
Ipswich	0473 704430	Direct Line
	or 0473 704431	Direct Line
Leeds	0532 430715	Direct Line
Leicester	0553 555779	Direct Line
Liverpool	051-236 4620	Extn 2126/2127/2128
London (Guy's Hospital)	071-955 5000	Extn 3594/5892
	or 071-378 0023	Direct Line
London (London Hospital)	071-377 7487	Direct Line
	or 071-377 7488	Direct Line
London (Northwick Park)	081-869 3973	Direct Line
Manchester	061-225 2063	Direct Line
	or 061-276 6270	Direct Line
Newcastle	091-232 1525	Direct Line
Oxford	0865 221808	Direct Line
	or 0865 221836	Direct Line
Southampton	0703 796908	Direct Line
	or 0703 796909	Direct Line

Northern Ireland		
Belfast	0232 248095	Direct Line
Londonderry	0504 45171	Extn 3262

Scotland		
Aberdeen	0224 681818	Extn 52316
Dundee	0382 60111	Extn 2351
Edinburgh	031-519 5482	Direct Line
	or 031-519 5454	Direct Line
Glasgow	041-552 4726	Direct Line
Inverness	0463 234151	Extn 288
	or 0463 220157	Direct Line

Wales		
Cardiff	0222 742979	Direct Line

Poisons Information Services

Belfast	0232 240503
Birmingham	021-554 3801
Cardiff	0222 709901
Dublin	Dublin 379964 or Dublin 379966
Edinburgh	031-229 2477
	or 031-228 2441 (Viewdata)
Leeds	0532 430715 or 0532 432799
London	071-635 9191 or 071-955 5095
Newcastle	091-232 5131

Note. Some of these centres also advise on laboratory analytical services which may be of help in the diagnosis and management of a small number of cases.

Pregnancy

Drugs can have harmful effects on the fetus at any time during pregnancy. Experience with many drugs in pregnancy is limited.

During the *first trimester* they may produce congenital malformations (teratogenesis), and the period of greatest risk is from the third to the eleventh week of pregnancy.

During the *second* and *third trimesters* drugs may affect the growth and functional development of the fetus or have toxic effects on fetal tissues; and drugs given shortly before term or during labour may have adverse effects on labour or on the neonate after delivery.

The following table lists drugs which may have harmful effects in pregnancy and indicates the trimester of risk.

The table is based on human data, but information on *animal* studies has been included for some newer drugs when its omission might be misleading.

Drugs should be prescribed in pregnancy only if the expected benefit to the mother is thought to be greater than the risk to the fetus, and all drugs should be avoided if possible during the first trimester. Drugs which have been extensively used in pregnancy and appear to be usually safe should be prescribed in preference to new or untried drugs; and the smallest effective dose should be used.

Few drugs have been shown conclusively to be teratogenic in man but no drug is safe beyond all doubt in early pregnancy. Screening procedures are available where there is a known risk of certain defects.

It should be noted that the BNF provides independent advice and may not always agree with the data sheets.

Absence of a drug from the list does not imply safety.

Table of drugs to be avoided or used with caution in pregnancy
Products introduced or amended since publication of BNF No. 24 (September 1992) are <u>underlined</u>

Drug (Trimester of risk)	Comments	Drug (Trimester of risk)	Comments
<u>ACE Inhibitors</u> (1, 2, 3)	Avoid; may adversely affect fetal and neonatal blood pressure control and renal function; also possible skull defects and oligohydrammios; toxicity in *animal* studies	Anaesthetics, Local (3)	With large doses, neonatal respiratory depression, hypotonia, and bradycardia after paracervical or epidural block; neonatal methaemoglobinaemia with prilocaine and procaine
Acebutolol see Beta-blockers		Analgesics see Opioid Analgesics and NSAIDs	
Acemetacin see NSAIDs		Androgens	Masculinisation of female
Acetazolamide see Diuretics		(1, 2, 3)	fetus
Acetohexamide see Sulphonylureas		Anistreplase see Streptokinase	
Acitretin see Etretinate		Anticoagulants	
Acrivastine see Antihistamines		Heparin	Osteoporosis has been
<u>Albendazole</u>	Manufacturer advises teratogenic in *animal* studies	(1, 2, 3)	reported after prolonged use
Alclometasone see Corticosteroids		Oral	Congenital malformations;
Alcohol		Anticoagulants	fetal and neonatal
(1, 2)	Regular daily drinking is teratogenic ('fetal alcohol syndrome') and may cause growth retardation; occasional single drinks are probably safe	(1, 2, 3)	haemorrhage *See also* section 2.8
		Antidepressants	
		MAOIs,	No evidence of harm but
		Serotonin-uptake	manufacturers advise avoid
		Inhibitor	unless compelling reasons
(3)	Withdrawal syndrome may occur in babies of alcoholic mothers	(1, 2, 3)	
		Tricyclic	Tachycardia, irritability,
		(and related)	muscle spasms, and
Alfentanil see Opioid Analgesics		(3)	convulsions in neonate reported occasionally
Allyloestrenol see Progestogens		Antiepileptics	Benefit of treatment
Alprazolam see Anxiolytics and Hypnotics			outweighs risk to fetus; risk
Alteplase see Streptokinase			of teratogenicity greater if
<u>Amantadine</u>	Toxicity in *animal* studies		more than one drug used;
Amikacin see Aminoglycosides			**important:** *see also*
Amiloride see Diuretics			carbamazepine,
Aminoglutethimide	Avoid; toxicity in *animal* studies and may affect fetal sexual development		ethosuximide, phenobarbitone, phenytoin, valproate, and section 4.8
Aminoglycosides	Auditory or vestibular nerve damage; risk greatest with steptomycin; probably very small with gentamicin and tobramycin	Antihistamines	No evidence of teratogenicity; some packs of antihistamines sold to the public carry warning to avoid in pregnancy; manufacturer of astemizole advises avoid (see p. 128)
(2, 3)			
Aminophylline see Theophylline			
Amiodarone	Possible risk of neonatal goitre; use only if no alternative	Antimalarials (1, 3)	Benefit of prophylaxis and treatment in malaria outweighs risk; **important:** *see also* individual drugs
(2, 3)			
Amitriptyline see Antidepressants, Tricyclic			
Amlodipine see Calcium-channel Blockers		Antipsychotics	Extrapyramidal effects in
Amoxapine see Antidepressants, Tricyclic		(3)	neonate occasionally reported
Amylobarbitone see Barbiturates		Anxiolytics and	Depress neonatal respiration.
Anabolic Steroids	Masculinisation of female	Hypnotics	Benzodiazepines cause
(1, 2, 3)	fetus	(3)	neonatal drowsiness,
Anaesthetics, General	Depress neonatal respiration		hypotonia, and withdrawal
(3)			

Drug (Trimester of risk)	Comments	Drug (Trimester of risk)	Comments
	symptoms; avoid large doses and regular use; short-acting benzodiazepines preferable to long-acting	Buserelin	Avoid
		Butriptyline *see* Antidepressants, Tricyclic	
		Calcium-channel Blockers	May inhibit labour and manufacturers advise that diltiazem and some dihydropyridines are teratogenic in *animals*
Aspirin (3)	Impaired platelet function and risk of haemorrhage; delayed onset and increased duration of labour with increased blood loss; avoid analgesic doses if possible in last week (low doses probably not harmful); with high doses, closure of fetal ductus arteriosus *in utero* and possibly persistent pulmonary hypertension of newborn; kernicterus in jaundiced neonates		
		Capreomycin	Manufacturer advises teratogenic in *animal* studies
		Captopril *see* ACE Inhibitors	
		Carbamazepine (1)	May be small risk of teratogenesis including increased risk of neural tube defects (screening advised); folate supplements should be given; *see also* Antiepileptics
		Carbenoxolone (3)	Avoid; causes sodium retention with oedema
Astemizole *see* Antihistamines		Carbimazole (2, 3)	Neonatal goitre and hypothyroidism. Has been associated with aplasia cutis of the neonate
Atenolol *see* Beta-blockers			
Auranofin *see* Gold			
Aurothiomalate *see* Gold			
Azapropazone *see* NSAIDs		Celiprolol *see* Beta-blockers	
Azatadine *see* Antihistamines		Cetirizine *see* Antihistamines	
Azathioprine *see* section 8.1		Chenodeoxycholic Acid (1, 2, 3)	Theoretical risk of effects on fetal metabolism
Azelastine *see* Antihistamines			
Aztreonam	Manufacturer advises avoid (but no evidence of teratogenicity)	Chloral hydrate *see* Anxiolytics and Hypnotics	
		Chloramphenicol (3)	Neonatal 'grey syndrome'
Barbiturates (3)	Withdrawal effects in neonate; *see also* Phenobarbitone	Chlordiazepoxide *see* Anxiolytics and Hypnotics	
		Chlormethiazole *see* Anxiolytics and Hypnotics	
		Chlormezanone *see* Anxiolytics and Hypnotics	
Beclomethasone *see* Corticosteroids		Chloroquine *see* Antimalarials	
Bendrofluazide *see* Diuretics		Chlorothiazide *see* Diuretics	
Benorylate [aspirin-paracetamol ester] *see* Aspirin		Chlorpheniramine *see* Antihistamines	
Benperidol *see* Antipsychotics		Chlorpromazine *see* Antipsychotics	
Benserazide [ingredient] *see Madopar®*		Chlorpropamide *see* Sulphonylureas	
Benzodiazepines *see* Anxiolytics and Hypnotics		Chlorprothixene *see* Antipsychotics	
Beta-blockers (3)	May cause intra-uterine growth retardation, neonatal hypoglycaemia, and bradycardia; risk greater in severe hypertension	Chlortetracycline *see* Tetracyclines	
		Chlorthalidone *see* Diuretics	
		Choline magnesium trisalicylate *see* Aspirin	
		Cilazapril *see* ACE Inhibitors	
Betamethasone *see* Corticosteroids		Cinnarizine *see* Antihistamines	
Betaxolol *see* Beta-blockers		Ciprofibrate *see* Clofibrate	
Bethanidine *see* Guanethidine		Ciprofloxacin *see* 4-Quinolones	
Bezafibrate *see* Clofibrate		Cisapride	Manufacturer advises avoid
Bisoprolol *see* Beta-blockers		Clemastine *see* Antihistamines	
Bisphosphonates	Manufacturers advise avoid (on theoretical grounds)	Clobazam *see* Anxiolytics and Hypnotics	
		Clobetasol *see* Corticosteroids	
Bromazepam *see* Anxiolytics and Hypnotics		Clobetasone *see* Corticosteroids	
Brompheniramine *see* Antihistamines		Clodronate sodium *see* Bisphosphonates	
Budesonide *see* Corticosteroids		Clofibrate (1, 2, 3)	Avoid—theoretical possibility of interference with embryonic growth and development due to anticholesterol effect
Bumetanide *see* Diuretics			
Bupivacaine *see* Anaesthetics, Local			
Buprenorphine *see* Opioid Analgesics			

Drug (Trimester of risk)	Comments	Drug (Trimester of risk)	Comments
Clomiphene	Possible effects on fetal development	Diazoxide (2, 3)	Prolonged use may produce alopecia and impaired glucose tolerance in neonate; inhibits uterine activity during labour
Clomipramine *see* Antidepressants, Tricyclic			
Clomocycline *see* Tetracyclines			
Clonazepam *see* Antiepileptics		Diclofenac *see* NSAIDs	
Clorazepate *see* Anxiolytics and Hypnotics		Diethylpropion	Avoid—congenital malformations reported to CSM
Clozapine	Manufacturer advises avoid		
Codeine *see* Opioid Analgesics			
Contraceptives, Oral	Epidemiological evidence suggests no harmful effects on fetus	Diflucortolone *see* Corticosteroids	
		Diflunisal *see* NSAIDs	
Corticosteroids (2, 3)	Benefit of treatment, e.g. in asthma, outweighs risk; high doses (>10 mg prednisolone daily) may produce fetal and neonatal adrenal suppression; corticosteroid cover required by mother during labour	Dihydrocodeine *see* Opioid Analgesics	
		Dihydroergotamine *see* Ergotamine	
		Diltiazem *see* Calcium-channel Blockers	
		Dimenhydrinate *see* Antihistamines	
		Dimethindene *see* Antihistamines	
		Diphenhydramine *see* Antihistamines	
		Diphenoxylate *see* Opioid Analgesics	
Co-trimoxazole		Diphenylpyraline *see* Antihistamines	
(1)	Possible teratogenic risk (trimethoprim a folate antagonist)	Dipipanone *see* Opioid Analgesics	
		Disodium Etidronate *see* Bisphosphonates	
		Disodium Pamidronate *see* Bisphosphonates	
(3)	Neonatal haemolysis and methaemoglobinaemia; fear of increased risk of kernicterus in neonates appears to be unfounded	Disopyramide (3)	May induce labour
		Distigmine	Manufacturer advises avoid (may stimulate uterine contractions)
Cyclizine *see* Antihistamines			
Cyclopenthiazide *see* Diuretics			
Cyclosporin *see* section 8.1		Disulfiram (1)	High concentrations of acetaldehyde which occur in presence of alcohol may be teratogenic
Cyproheptadine *see* Antihistamines			
Cyproterone [ingredient] *see* Dianette®			
Cytotoxic drugs (1)	Most are teratogenic; see section 8.1	Diuretics (3)	Not used to treat hypertension in pregnancy; thiazides may cause neonate thrombocytopenia
Danazol (1, 2, 3)	Has weak androgenic effects and virilisation of female fetus reported		
		Dothiepin *see* Antidepressants, Tricyclic	
Dapsone (3)	Neonatal haemolysis and methaemoglobinaemia; folate supplements should be given to mother	Doxepin *see* Antidepressants, Tricyclic	
		Doxycycline *see* Tetracyclines	
		Droperidol *see* Antipsychotics	
		Dydrogesterone *see* Progestogens	
Debrisoquine *see* Guanethidine		Enalapril *see* ACE Inhibitors	
Demeclocycline *see* Tetracyclines		Enflurane *see* Anaesthetics, General	
Desferrioxamine	Manufacturer advises toxicity in *animal* studies	Ergotamine (1, 2, 3)	Oxytocic effects on the pregnant uterus
Desipramine *see* Antidepressants, Tricyclic		Esmolol *see* Beta-blockers	
Desonide *see* Corticosteroids		Ethacrynic acid *see* Diuretics	
Desoxymethasone *see* Corticosteroids		Ether *see* Anaesthetics, General	
Dexamethasone *see* Corticosteroids		Ethinyloestradiol *see* Contraceptives, Oral	
Dextromethorphan *see* Opioid Analgesics		Ethionamide (1)	May be teratogenic
Dextromoramide *see* Opioid Analgesics			
Dextropropoxyphene *see* Opioid Analgesics		Ethosuximide (1)	May possibly be teratogenic *see* Antiepileptics
Diamorphine *see* Opioid Analgesics			
Dianette® (1, 2, 3)	Feminisation of male fetus (due to cyproterone)	Etidronate Disodium *see* Bisphosphonates	
		Etodolac *see* NSAIDs	
Diazepam *see* Anxiolytics and Hypnotics		Etomidate *see* Anaesthetics, General	

Drug (Trimester of risk)	Comments	Drug (Trimester of risk)	Comments
Etretinate (1, 2, 3)	Teratogenic; effective contraception must be used for at least 1 month before treatment, during treatment and for at least two years after stopping	Gliclazide see Sulphonylureas	
		Glipizide see Sulphonylureas	
		Gliquidone see Sulphonylureas	
		Gold	
		Auranofin	Manufacturer advises teratogenicity in animal studies; effective contraception should be used during and for at least 6 months after treatment
Fansidar® (1)	Possible teratogenic risk (pyrimethamine a folate antagonist)		
(3)	Neonatal haemolysis and methaemoglobinaemia; fear of increased risk of kernicterus in neonates appears to be unfounded see also Antimalarials	Aurothiomalate (1, 2, 3)	No good evidence of harm but avoid if possible
		Griseofulvin	CRM advises avoid (fetotoxicity and teratogenicity in animals)
Felodipine see Calcium-channel Blockers		Growth Hormone	Avoid on theoretical grounds
Fenbufen see NSAIDs		Guanethidine (3)	Postural hypotension and reduced uteroplacental perfusion; should not be used to treat hypertension in pregnancy
Fenofibrate (1, 2, 3)	Manufacturer advises toxicity in animal studies; see also Clofibrate		
Fenoprofen see NSAIDs		Halcinonide see Corticosteroids	
Fentanyl see Opioid Analgesics		Halofantrine (1)	Manufacturer advises teratogenicity in animal studies
Finasteride (1, 2, 3)	Avoid unprotected intercourse (see section 6.4.2). May cause feminisation of male fetus		
		Haloperidol see Antipsychotics	
		Halothane see Anaesthetics, General	
Flecainide	Manufacturer advises toxicity in animal studies	Heparin see Anticoagulants	
		Hydralazine (1)	Manufacturer advises toxicity in animal studies
Fluclorolone see Corticosteroids			
Fluconazole	Manufacturer advises toxicity at high doses in animal studies	Hydrochlorothiazide see Diuretics	
		Hydrocortisone see Corticosteroids	
		Hydroflumethiazide see Diuretics	
Flucytosine (1)	Possible teratogenic risk	Hydroxychloroquine Avoid for rheumatic disease (but for malaria see Antimalarials)	
Flunitrazepam see Anxiolytics and Hypnotics			
Fluocinolone see Corticosteroids		Hydroxyprogesterone see Progestogens	
Fluocinomide see Corticosteroids		Hydroxyzine see Antihistamines	
Fluocortolone see Corticosteroids		Hypnotics see Anxiolytics and Hypnotics	
Fluoxetine see Antidepressants		Ibuprofen see NSAIDs	
Flupenthixol see Antipsychotics		Idoxuridine	Manufacturers advise toxicity in animal studies
Fluphenazine see Antipsychotics			
Flurandrenolone see Corticosteroids		Imipramine see Antidepressants, Tricyclic	
Flurazepam see Anxiolytics and Hypnotics		Immunosuppressants see section 8.1	
Flurbiprofen see NSAIDs		Indapamide see Diuretics	
Fluspirilene see Antipsychotics		Indomethacin see NSAIDs	
Fluvoxamine see Antidepressants		Interferons	Manufacturers recommend avoid unless compelling reasons; not for chronic active hepatitis during pregnancy
Foscarnet	Manufacturer advises avoid		
Fosinopril see ACE Inhibitors			
Frusemide see Diuretics			
Ganciclovir	Avoid—teratogenic risk	Iodine and Iodides (2, 3)	Neonatal goitre and hypothyroidism
Gemfibrozil see Clofibrate			
Gentamicin see Aminoglycosides		Radioactive iodine (1, 2, 3)	Permanent hypothyroidism— avoid
Gestrinone (1, 2, 3)	Avoid		
Glibenclamide see Sulphonylureas		Iprindole see Antidepressants, Tricyclic (and related)	

Drug (Trimester of risk)	Comments	Drug (Trimester of risk)	Comments
Isoflurane see Anaesthetics, General		Mebendazole	Manufacturer advises toxicity in *animal* studies
Isotretinoin (1, 2, 3)	Teratogenic; effective contraception must be used for at least 1 month before oral treatment, during treatment and for at least 1 month after stopping; also avoid topical treatment	Mebhydrolin see Antihistamines	
		Medazepam see Anxiolytics and Hypnotics	
		Mefenamic Acid see NSAIDs	
		Mefloquine (1)	Manufacturer advises teratogenicity in *animal* studies; avoid for prophylaxis, see p. 247
Isoxsuprine	For cautions on use in uncomplicated premature labour see section 7.1.3		
		Mefruside see Diuretics	
Isradipine see Calcium-channel Blockers		Meprobamate see Anxiolytics and Hypnotics	
Itraconazole	Manufacturer advises toxicity in *animal* studies	Meptazinol see Opioid Analgesics	
		Mesterolone see Androgens	
Kanamycin see Aminoglycosides		Mestranol see Contraceptives, Oral	
Ketamine see Anaesthetics, General		Metaraminol (1, 2, 3)	Avoid—may reduce placental perfusion
Ketoconazole	Manufacturer advises teratogenicity in *animal* studies; packs carry a warning to avoid in pregnancy	Metformin (1, 2, 3)	Avoid
		Methadone see Opioid Analgesics	
		Methohexitone see Anaesthetics, General	
Ketoprofen see NSAIDs		Methotrimeprazine see Antipsychotics	
Ketorolac see NSAIDs		Methyclothiazide see Diuretics	
Ketotifen see Antihistamines		Methylphenobarbitone see Antiepileptics	
Labetalol see Beta-blockers		Methylprednisolone see Corticosteroids	
Lamotrigine see Antiepileptics		Metolazone see Diuretics	
Levodopa	Manufacturers advise toxicity in *animal* studies	Metroprolol see Beta-blockers	
		Metronidazole	Manufacturer advises avoidance of high-dose regimens
Lignocaine see Anaesthetics, Local			
Lindane	Manufacturer advises toxicity in *animal* studies	Metyrapone	Avoid (may impair biosynthesis of fetal-placental steroids)
Lisinopril see ACE Inhibitors			
Lithium (1, 2, 3)	Dose requirements increased; congenital malformations; neonatal goitre reported; lithium toxicity (hypotonia and cyanosis) in neonate if maternal therapy poorly controlled	Mianserin see Antidepressants, Tricyclic (and related)	
		Mifepristone	Manufacturer advises that if treatment fails, essential that pregnancy be terminated by another method
		Minocycline see Tetracyclines	
Lofepramine see Antidepressants, Tricyclic		Minoxidil (3)	Neonatal hirsutism reported
Loprazolam see Anxiolytics and Hypnotics		Misoprostol (1, 2, 3)	Avoid; increases uterine tone
Loratadine see Antihistamines			
Lorazepam see Anxiolytics and Hypnotics		Molgramostim	Manufacturer advises toxicity in *animal* studies
Lormetazepam see Anxiolytics and Hypnotics			
Lymecycline see Tetracyclines		Morphine see Opioid Analgesics	
Madopar® see Levodopa		Nabumetone see NSAIDs	
Maloprim®		Nadolol see Beta-blockers	
(1)	Possible teratogenic risk (pyrimethamine a folate antagonist)	Nafarelin	Avoid
		Nalbuphine see Opioid Analgesics	
		Nalidixic acid see 4-Quinolones	
(3)	Neonatal haemolysis and methaemoglobinaemia (due to dapsone); folate supplements should be given to mother see also Antimalarials	Nandrolone see Anabolic Steroids	
		Naproxen see NSAIDs	
		Narcotic Analgesics see Opioid Analgesics	
		Neomycin see Aminoglycosides	
		Neostigmine (3)	Neonatal myasthenia with large doses
Maprotiline see Antidepressants, Tricyclic (and related)			

258 • Appendix 2: Drugs and pregnancy

Drug (Trimester of risk)	Comments
Netilmicin see Aminoglycosides	
Nicardipine see Calcium-channel Blockers	
Nicoumalone see Anticoagulants	
Nifedipine see Calcium-channel Blockers	
Nimodipine see Calcium-channel Blockers	
Nitrazepam see Anxiolytics and Hypnotics	
Nitrofurantoin (3)	May produce neonatal haemolysis if used at term
Nitrous oxide see Anaesthetics, General	
Noradrenaline (1, 2, 3)	Avoid—may reduce placental perfusion
Norfloxacin see 4-Quinolones	
Nortriptyline see Antidepressants, Tricyclic	
NSAIDs (3)	With regular use closure of fetal ductus arteriosus in utero and possibly persistent pulmonary hypertension of the newborn. Delayed onset and increased duration of labour
Octreotide (1, 2, 3)	Avoid; possible effect on fetal growth
Oestrogens see Contraceptives, Oral	
Ofloxacin see 4-Quinolones	
Omeprazole	Manufacturer advises toxicity in animal studies
Opioid Analgesics (1)	Avoid papaveretum (contains noscapine which may be teratogenic)
(3)	Depress neonatal respiration; withdrawal effects in neonates of dependent mothers; gastric stasis and risk of inhalation pneumonia in mother during labour
Oxatomide see Antihistamines	
Oxazepam see Anxiolytics and Hypnotics	
Oxprenolol see Beta-blockers	
Oxybutynin	Manufacturer advises toxicity at high doses in animal studies
Oxymetholone see Anabolic Steroids	
Oxypertine see Antipsychotics	
Oxytetracycline see Tetracyclines	
Pamidronate Disodium see Bisphosphonates	
Papaveretum see Opioid Analgesics	
Paroxetine see Antidepressants	
Penbutolol see Beta-blockers	
Penicillamine (1, 2, 3)	Fetal abnormalities reported rarely; avoid if possible
Pentazocine see Opioid Analgesics	
Pericyazine see Antipsychotics	
Perindopril see ACE Inhibitors	
Perphenazine see Antipsychotics	
Pethidine see Opioid Analgesics	

Drug (Trimester of risk)	Comments
Phenindamine see Antihistamines	
Phenindione see Anticoagulants	
Pheniramine see Antihistamines	
Phenobarbitone (1, 3)	Congenital malformations. Neonatal bleeding tendency—prophylactic vitamin K₁ should be given; see also Antiepileptics
Phenoperidine see Opioid Analgesics	
Phenothiazines see Antipsychotics	
Phenytoin (1, 3)	Congenital malformations (screening advised). Folate supplements should be given to mother (reduced absorption). Neonatal bleeding tendency—prophylactic vitamin K₁ should be given. Caution in interpreting plasma concentrations—bound may be reduced but free (i.e. effective) unchanged; see also Antiepileptics
Pholcodine see Opioid Analgesics	
Pimozide see Antipsychotics	
Pindolol see Beta-blockers	
Piperazine	No clinical evidence of harm but packs sold to the general public carry a warning to avoid in pregnancy except on medical advice
Pipothiazine see Antipsychotics	
Piroxicam see NSAIDs	
Podophyllum resin (1, 2, 3)	Avoid—neonatal death and teratogenesis have been reported
Polythiazide see Diuretics	
Povidone-iodine (2, 3)	Sufficient iodine may be absorbed to affect the fetal thyroid
Pravastatin see Clofibrate	
Prednisolone see Corticosteroids	
Prednisone see Corticosteroids	
Prilocaine (3)	Neonatal methaemo-globinaemia; see also Anaesthetics, Local
Primaquine (3)	Neonatal haemolysis and methaemoglobinaemia; see also Antimalarials
Primidone see Antiepileptics	
Probucol see Clofibrate	
Procaine (3)	Neonatal methaemoglobinaemia; see also Anaesthetics, Local
Prochlorperazine see Antipsychotics	

Drug (Trimester of risk)	Comments	Drug (Trimester of risk)	Comments
Progestogens (1)	High doses may possibly be teratogenic	Stanozolol see Anabolic Steroids	
Proguanil	Folate supplements should be given to mother; see also Antimalarials	Stilboestrol (1)	High doses associated with vaginal carcinoma, urogenital abnormalities, and reduced fertility in female offspring
Promazine see Antipsychotics		Streptokinase (1, 2, 3)	Possibility of premature separation of placenta in first 18 weeks; theoretical possibility of fetal haemorrhage throughout pregnancy; avoid postpartum use—maternal haemorrhage
Promethazine see Antihistamines			
Propofol see Anaesthetics, General			
Propranolol see Beta-blockers			
Propylthiouracil (2, 3)	Neonatal goitre and hypothyroidism		
Prothionamide (1)	May be teratogenic	Streptomycin see Aminoglycosides	
Protriptyline see Antidepressants, Tricyclic		Sulfadoxine see Sulphonamides	
Pyridostigmine (3)	Neonatal myasthenia with large doses	Sulfametopyrazine see Sulphonamides	
Pyrimethamine (1)	Possible teratogenic risk (folate antagonist); folate supplements should be given to mother; see also Antimalarials	Sulindac see NSAIDs	
		Sulphadiazine see Sulphonamides	
		Sulphadimidine see Sulphonamides	
		Sulphasalazine (3)	Theoretical risk of neonatal haemolysis; folate supplements should be given to mother
Quinapril see ACE Inhibitors			
Quinine (1)	High doses are teratogenic but in malaria benefit of treatment outweighs risk	Sulphonamides (3)	Neonatal haemolysis and methaemoglobinaemia; fear of increased risk of kernicterus in neonates appears to be unfounded
4-Quinolones (1, 2, 3)	Arthropathy in animal studies		
Ramipril see ACE Inhibitors		Sulphonylureas (3)	Neonatal hypoglycaemia; insulin is normally substituted in all diabetics; if oral drugs are used therapy should be stopped at least 2 days before delivery
Remoxipride see Antipsychotics			
Rifampicin (1)	Manufacturers advise very high doses teratogenic in animal studies		
(3)	Risk of neonatal bleeding may be increased	Sulpiride see Antipsychotics	
		Tamoxifen	Possible effects on fetal development
Ritodrine	For cautions on use in uncomplicated premature labour see section 7.1.3	Temazepam see Anxiolytics and Hypnotics	
		Tenoxicam see NSAIDs	
		Terbutaline see Salbutamol	
Salbutamol (3)	Large parenteral doses given at term for asthma could delay onset of labour; risk ketoacidosis in diabetic women; for cautions on use in uncomplicated premature labour see section 7.1.3	Terfenadine see Antihistamines	
		Testosterone see Androgens	
		Tetracyclines (2, 3)	Dental discoloration; maternal hepatotoxicity with large parenteral doses
		Theophylline (3)	Neonatal irritability and apnoea have been reported
Salicylates see Aspirin		Thiabendazole (1)	Teratogenic in animal studies
Salsalate see Aspirin			
Sertraline see Antidepressants			
Simvastatin	Manufacturer advises toxicity in animal studies	Thiazides (3)	May cause neonatal thrombocytopenia; see also Diuretics
Sodium Aurothiomalate see Gold			
Sodium Clodronate see Bisphosphonates		Thiethylperazine see Antipsychotics	
Sodium Valproate see Valproate		Thiopentone see Anaesthetics, General	
Sotalol see Beta-blockers		Thioridazine see Antipsychotics	
Spironolactone	Manufacturers advise toxicity in animal studies	Tiaprofenic Acid see NSAIDs	
		Timolol see Beta-blockers	

Drug (Trimester of risk)	Comments	Drug (Trimester of risk)	Comments
Tinidazole	Manufacturer advises avoid in first trimester	(1, 2, 3)	separation of placenta in first 18 weeks; theoretical possibility of fetal haemorrhage throughout pregnancy; avoid postpartum use—maternal haemorrhage
Tobramycin *see* Aminoglycosides			
Tocainide	Manufacturer advises toxicity in *animal* studies		
Tolbutamide *see* Sulphonylureas		Vaccines (live)	Theoretical risk of congenital malformations; see section 14.1
Tolmetin *see* NSAIDs		(1)	
Trazodone *see* Antidepressants, Tricyclic (and related)			
Tretinoin	Avoid; other retinoids teratogenic	Valproate (1, 3)	Increased risk of neural tube defects (screening advised); neonatal bleeding and hepatotoxicity also reported; *see also* Antiepileptics
Triamcinolone *see* Corticosteroids			
Triamterene *see* Diuretics			
Tribavirin	Manufacturer advises avoid		
Triclofos *see* Anxiolytics and Hypnotics		Verapamil *see* Calcium-channel Blockers	
Trifluoperazine *see* Antipsychotics		Vigabatrin	Manufacturer advises toxicity in *animal* studies; *see also* Antiepileptics
Trifluperidol *see* Antipsychotics			
Trilostane (1, 2, 3)	Interferes with placental sex hormone production		
Trimeprazine *see* Antihistamines		Viloxazine *see* Antidepressants, Tricyclic (and related)	
Trimetaphan (3)	Avoid. Risk of paralytic ileus in newborn	Vitamin A (1)	Excessive doses may be teratogenic; *see also* p. 357
Trimethoprim (1)	Possible teratogenic risk (folate antagonist)	Warfarin *see* Anticoagulants	
Trimipramine *see* Antidepressants, Tricyclic		Xamoterol	Manufacturer advises toxicity in *animal* studies
Triprolidine *see* Antihistamines		Xipamide *see* Diuretics	
Urokinase	Possibility of premature	Zuclopenthixol *see* Antipsychotics	

Index

Bold type indicates illustrations